Artificial Intelligence-Enabled Security for Healthcare Systems

Sunil Gupta • Monit Kapoor
Sanjoy Kumar Debnath

Artificial Intelligence-Enabled Security for Healthcare Systems

Safeguarding Patient Data and Improving Services

Springer

Sunil Gupta
School of Computer Science
University of Petroleum and Energy
Dehradun, Uttarakhand, India

Sanjoy Kumar Debnath
Chitkara University Institute of Engineering
and Technology, Chitkara University
Rajpura, Punjab, India

Monit Kapoor
Department of Computer Science
and Engineering
Amity School of Engineering and
Technology, Amity University
Bengaluru, Karnataka, India

ISBN 978-3-031-82809-6 ISBN 978-3-031-82810-2 (eBook)
https://doi.org/10.1007/978-3-031-82810-2

This Springer imprint is published by the registered company Springer Nature Switzerland AG
The registered company address is: Gewerbestrasse 11, 6330 Cham, Switzerland

Foreword

Artificial intelligence has impacted every discipline in modern times by helping to solve many problems in various sectors and domains. Healthcare sector has been deeply impacted by the usage of AI in recent times, as it has led to creation of faster and more accurate set of healthcare services for patients in the area of monitoring, diagnostics and treatment of ailments. However, usage of AI has thrown up unique challenges like security and privacy of patient data, vulnerability of data and possible data breaches. Therefore, safeguarding patient interests and ensuring their privacy and safety is of utmost importance and needs to be ensured at all levels and under all circumstances.

The present book, titled *Artificial Intelligence-Enabled Security for Healthcare Systems: Safeguarding Patient Data and Improving Services*, is a timely attempt to address pressing issues around data privacy and security issues for patient-centric information and maintain quality of service while addressing the concerns posed by adoption of security mechanisms while handling patient data and providing patient-centric services while using Artificial Intelligence. The authors have tried to address issues like security and privacy of patient information, quality service mechanisms and combination of AI and security in healthcare in a lucid and engaging manner. The authors have written ten chapters in a chronological manner starting from introduction to the domain of AI and security in healthcare, security solutions in AI-led healthcare delivery mechanisms, Analytics for healthcare, best practices in healthcare industry enabled by AI and case studies, and the book culminates with future direction of work in this prominent area of healthcare coupled with AI and security challenges.

The overall selection of topics and titles for chapters and the organization of all chapters have been done in a manner that readers will find them very engaging and interesting. The chapters have been illustrated with sufficient tabulated information, diagrams and pictures and comparative charts wherever necessary. The authors have touched upon every aspect of healthcare, analytics, security, privacy issues and patient centricity in healthcare while authoring these ten very well-written chapters. I am very sure that the book will be well received in academic circles and would enjoy high readership amongst research scholars, academicians, UG and PG students and practitioners alike. All the chapters are sufficient in details and have been written in a concise manner, elaborating upon all necessary factors of the domain of security in AI led healthcare systems. The chapters have shed enough focus on research issues for each topic. I congratulate the authors for their attempt to write on such a relevant and important topic that concerns humanity in our present times. I also congratulate the Springer Nature group to have collaborated on this very timely book project. I convey my best wishes to all authors and readers of this book alike and I am sure the community shall keep on writing about this important area in future as well.

Vice Chancellor, Amity University
Bengaluru, Karnataka, India
D. Subhakar

Preface

In an era where healthcare systems are increasingly reliant on digital infrastructure, the integration of artificial intelligence (AI) has emerged as a transformative force, enhancing efficiency, improving patient outcomes, and expanding the capabilities of healthcare providers. Yet, alongside these benefits come significant challenges, particularly regarding the security and privacy of sensitive patient data. As healthcare systems adopt AI-based technologies to reinforce their services, the need for robust security solutions has become paramount. This book, *Artificial Intelligence-Enabled Security for Healthcare Systems: Safeguarding Patient Data and Improving Services,* examines the essential role AI plays in securing healthcare systems against growing cybersecurity threats.

The book begins with an exploration of AI's role in healthcare security and privacy in Chap. 1, setting the foundation by emphasizing the importance of safeguarding patient data and discussing how AI contributes to healthcare improvements. Following this, Chap. 2 introduces sensor-based Internet of Things (IoT) technologies, integral to modern healthcare systems, examining both the benefits and security challenges these technologies present.

Chapter 3 provides a thorough overview of cybersecurity risks and threats unique to healthcare, including case studies of high-profile cyber incidents that underline the impact of such attacks on patient care and healthcare organizations. To counter these challenges, Chap. 4 discusses current AI-based cybersecurity solutions, comparing their benefits and showcasing real-world implementations.

Recognizing the role of analytics, Chap. 5 illustrates how AI, through machine learning algorithms and predictive analytics, can strengthen cybersecurity measures in healthcare. Chapter 6 then addresses the inherent risks and challenges in implementing AI-enabled security, such as regulatory compliance, ethical considerations, and privacy concerns, offering strategic approaches to mitigate these issues.

Chapter 7 outlines best practices for the implementation of AI-enabled healthcare security, with a focus on integrating these solutions into existing healthcare systems while ensuring compliance with privacy and security standards. Building upon this, Chap. 8 discusses the potential positive impact of AI-enabled security on patient outcomes, highlighting successful implementations that have led to enhanced patient care and reduced data breach risks.

Looking ahead, Chap. 9 identifies emerging trends and technologies, exploring future possibilities and challenges in advancing AI-enabled healthcare security. Finally, Chap. 10 summarizes the book's key takeaways and offers recommendations for future research and practical advancements in this critical field.

This book is designed for healthcare professionals, security specialists, researchers, and policymakers who are navigating the evolving landscape of healthcare security. We hope it serves as a valuable resource, inspiring innovations that ensure healthcare systems are equipped to protect patient data while leveraging AI for enhanced care and service delivery.

Dehradun, Uttarakhand, India — Sunil Gupta

Bengaluru, Karnataka, India — Monit Kapoor

Rajpura, Punjab, India — Sanjoy Kumar Debnath

Contents

Chapter 1
Introduction to AI and Privacy Issues for Healthcare Systems

Contents

Abstract Artificial intelligence is a relatively new technology that is transforming healthcare through advanced diagnostics, personalized treatments, and efficient care of patients. However, the integration of AI into health care systems raises significant privacy and ethical concerns. In this chapter, an introduction to the very basics of AI and its applications to health care are presented, with emphasis on both the pros and cons of AI-driven solutions. We look at issues of privacy, security, and consent although limited in scope here and bias within AI algorithms applied to health. This is followed by a review of regulatory frameworks and best practice in ensuring that AI is applied ethically in healthcare. Artificial intelligence is increasingly used in health systems and applications, and questions and debates concerned with ethical issues and risks to privacy are underway. This paper has surveyed and discussed some of the ethical challenges, privacy risks, and possible solutions in safeguarding user data privacy in AI-enabled healthcare applications.

Keywords Artificial intelligence · Medical innovation · Diagnostic imaging · Predictive analytics · Personalised medicine · Data protection · Algorithmic bias · Privacy-preserving AI

S. Gupta et al., *Artificial Intelligence-Enabled Security for Healthcare Systems*,
https://doi.org/10.1007/978-3-031-82810-2_1

1.1 Introduction

AI has now joined the ranks of other forces of transformation that impact industries, and healthcare is no different. AI technologies can redefine the healthcare landscape in a gamut of ways, such as more accurate diagnostics, better, more personalized treatment plans, and improved care. The demands of the healthcare industry are on a rise in efficiency, precision, and scalability; in this respect, AI has promises on offer.

AI, at the very core, is the simulation of human intelligence processes by machines, especially computer systems that are engaged in these processes. The computers are made to learn by themselves from experiences, hence acquiring information and rules about several ways to use that information. In turn, that learning is used in reasoning to approximate or reach definite conclusions and then to finally self-correct. Technologies associated with AI in healthcare may, however, be roughly sorted into some key types, which vary in their capabilities and applications.

Machine Learning (ML) Machine learning is a subdomain of artificial intelligence that deals with developing algorithms that can allow computers to learn from and make predictions or decisions based on that learning. Machine learning in health means the analysis of complex medical data to identify patterns and provide insights that will help in diagnosis and treatment. One example is the use of ML algorithms to process large volumes of medical images for abnormalities; predict the advancement of the disease; and offer personalized treatment plans, based on the patient's data.

Natural Language Processing (NLP) This is the ability of a computer program to understand and comprehend human language as written and spoken. The functionality of NLP in health systems allows them an interpretation and generation of human language, which helps in deriving useful insights mainly from clinical notes, literature, and patient records. This is very important in such applications as automated transcription of doctor-patient interactions, sentiment analysis, and synthesis of patient information into concise, actionable insights.

Computer Vision Computer vision refers to the part of AI that allows computers to view and understand the real world physically and then act based on that understanding. Computer vision is applied in diagnostic imaging within healthcare. This follows automated analyses of medical images like X-rays, CT scans, and MRIs. It also offers support in places where radiologists can use computer-aided diagnosis to locate abnormalities more efficiently and effectively, hence improving diagnosis for the better care of patients.

Robotics and Automation Robotics in healthcare mimics human behaviour through Artificial Intelligence to achieve tasks accurately and precisely, repeatedly. For example, surgical robots assist surgeons during complex procedures with much more accuracy and are minimally invasive. AI-driven automation has also eased administrative tasks in healthcare, like appointment scheduling, billing, and management of patient data. This reduces the workload of healthcare professionals and makes the operations much smoother.

Expert Systems Expert systems are the AI programs that tend to imitate the human expert's decision-making ability. An Expert System is defined as a computer program designed to make decisions or solve problems in a particular domain using knowledge and reasoning methods like a human expert. The system uses a knowledge base of human experience, together with an inference engine, to reason through bodies of knowledge and solve complex problems. Such a system can support clinical decision-making in health care.

Integration of AI in evolving advanced healthcare systems testifies two ends of the spectrum: there would be opportunities and challenges. On the one hand, AI can be harnessed to revolutionize patient care, improve efficiency, and cut costs. On the other hand, the adoption of AI will raise critical concerns over data privacy, ethics, and the need for robust regulatory frameworks. This chapter explains the fundamental aspects of AI in healthcare, associated with its transformative potential and complex problems in its application. We seek to move the discussion forward by explicating a nuanced understanding of how AI can shape the future of health through a comprehensive exploration of AI technologies and applications.

1.2 Overview of AI Applications in Healthcare

Artificial Intelligence opens a new age in the health sector through innovation of solutions to improve patient outcomes, smoothening operations, and raising the quality of care delivered. Applications of artificial intelligence in health systems have dramatically improved aspects related to diagnostic imaging, predictive analytics, and personalized medicine. Key applications are discussed herein regarding how AI technologies reshape healthcare.

1. Diagnostic Imaging:

AI is revolutionizing the accuracy and efficiency of image analysis in diagnostic imaging. Diagnostic imaging has traditionally been heavily dependent on radiologists and other medical professionals to make sense of the enormous number of complex images produced by tests such as X-rays, MRIs, and CT scans. Indeed, AI-based tools, especially those applied to deep learning and computer vision, can analyse effortlessly these images with a precision that often eludes the human eye.

Higher Accuracy AI algorithms can be trained on vast datasets of medical images to learn the trends and anomalies that associate specific diseases with certain trends and anomalies, increasing diagnosis accuracy and allowing for the early detection of conditions like cancer, cardiovascular diseases, and neurological disorders.

Increased Efficiency AI-driven diagnostic tools can process large volumes of images rapidly, thereby bringing down considerably the time required for analysis, which enables professionals to spend more time on other critical tasks and make informed decisions much faster.

Support to Radiologists AI does not replace radiologists; rather, it complements the ability of radiologists to provide additional insights and give them a second opinion in decision-making. Such collaboration between AI and health professionals improves diagnosis confidence and supports more accurate clinical decisions.

2. Predictive Analytics:

Predictive analytics uses AI to review past and real-time information to provide an ability to ascertain what will happen in the future, with time-sensitive interventions, make decisions informed by data. It plays a great role in predicting disease outbreaks, patient admission rates, and individual health trajectories.

Disease Prediction AI can analyse patient data, including such factors as medical history, lifestyle, and genetics, to provide the likelihood of certain conditions. Such a predictive capacity is allowing for early interventions and preventive measures to reduce the risks of progressing diseases.

Patient Risk Stratification The predictive analytics enables the identification of high-risk patients who require intensive monitoring and care. By stratifying patients according to their risk profiles, healthcare providers are better equipped to allocate resources and deliver the right interventions.

Operational Efficiency AI-driven predictive analytics helps hospitals smoothen their operations in terms of admission and resource prediction. In such optimization, healthcare facilities are effectively staffed and equipped to take care of patients; hence, improving the general efficiency by cutting down costs.

3. Personalized Medicine:

It applies individually with specific features, which is thus different from the application of the one-size-fits-all strategy in medical treatment. AI plays a very important role in accomplishing the practicality of personalized medicine by analysing various sources of data, such as genomic, clinical, and lifestyle information, to come up with bespoke treatment plans for individuals.

Genomic Analysis AI algorithms can process and interpret complex genomic data to identify genetic mutations and biomarkers for specific diseases. This kind of analysis permits the development of therapies targeted at the very genetic causes at the root of a condition, hence leading to the formation of more effective treatments.

Treatment Optimization AI would help analyse patient responses to various treatments, enabling health providers to identify the most effective interventions for patients. Optimization through the elimination of guesswork avoids several undesirable consequences and improves outcomes in patients.

Drug Discovery AI hastens the process of drug discovery by trawling large datasets for potential drug candidates and prediction of their efficacy and safety. This accelerates the development of new treatments and therapies on the market.

AI health care applications are designed to enhance diagnostic accuracy, create room for proactive interventions, and facilitate patient care as shown in Fig. 1.1. Advantages associated with these developments are also credited for several challenges: data privacy concerns, ethical dilemmas, and the requirement of an ideal

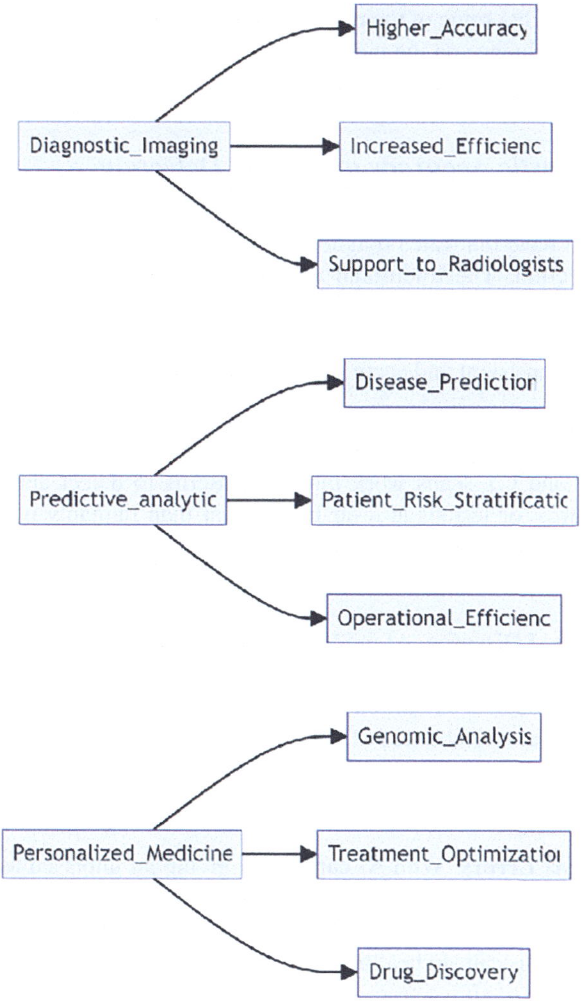

Fig. 1.1 AI application in healthcare

regulatory framework. For AI to really benefit the care of patients and advance innovation in the sector, it becomes very important that healthcare providers understand these challenges and know how to overcome them.

1.3 Benefits of AI in Healthcare

Artificial intelligence can be integrated into the healthcare systems to bring vast improvements in patient outcomes, diagnostic accuracy, and operational efficiency. Artificial intelligence in health will mostly help health professionals deliver accurate and personalized care, reduce costs, and speed up administrative operations. The section highlights some of the major benefits AI has brought to healthcare, noting its breakout influence on the industry.

1.3.1 Diagnostic Accuracy and Early Detection

AI technologies have innovated diagnosis, hence making it more accurate and fast in disease detection. The traditional diagnostic methods are mostly subjective-interpretive, placing the medical professional at the core of determination; hence, accuracy varies. AI, with its technologies of machine learning and computer vision, delivers a more consistent and accurate way of diagnosis.

Advanced Image Analysis AI-driven technology can do the analysis of medical images with a high degree of accuracy. For example, deep learning algorithms in X-rays, MRIs, and CT scans work through patterns to detect abnormalities like tumours, fractures, or lesions at a far better level than humanly possible. Indeed, some studies have proven that AI alone can rival, if not outperform, human expertise in the diagnosis of certain conditions like breast cancer seen in mammograms.

Early Detection of Diseases AI models can detect minute changes in medical data that may point at the beginning of diseases long before symptoms materialize. This becomes very critical in conditions such as cancer, where early intervention is paramount to increasing chances of survival. For example, genetic and molecular data analysed by AI algorithms project the probabilities of development of diseases so that preventive measures and early treatments can be administered.

Fewer Diagnosis Errors With AI capable of giving an unbiased assessment, the diagnostic errors are enormously reduced. In particular, it is highly useful in cases where various different conditions can share symptoms but have vastly different causes. Such AI tools can aid healthcare professionals by offering more insights and supporting findings to afford more accurate diagnoses.

1.3.2 Improved Care and Treatment Outcomes

The ability of AI to process large amounts of data and give relevant insights is a massive contribution toward better care and treatment. It helps health providers to deliver more effective and efficient services by personalization of treatment plans and optimization of clinical decision-making.

Personalized Treatment Plans By considering genetic, clinical, and lifestyle data specific to a patient, AI can collect and analyze them in order to come up with treatment plans personalized to better suit each case and increase chances of success. It is the kind of approach that will ensure all patients receive therapies most appropriate to them, based on their unique profiles, hence better outcomes and reduced side effects.

Predictive Analytics for Better Care Prediction by AI-powered predictive analytics can project patients' health trajectories in advance for interventions and timely care. For example, AI models would be able to predict a complication or readmission; hence, healthcare providers can take preventive measures and adjust treatment plans accordingly.

Optimized Clinical Decision-Making AI tools can help the clinicians make more informed decisions by providing them with evidence-based recommendations and indicating possible ways of treatment for patient conditions. Support of this nature allows healthcare professionals to broaden their range of possibilities in making data-backed decisions for better patient care.

Continuous Monitoring and Support AI-powered wearable devices, along with remote monitoring systems, track patients' continuous health metrics, such as heart rate, blood pressure, or glucose levels. In this way, real-time data is obtained that allows for timely interventions or changes in treatment plans, hence elevating patient safety and outcome.

1.3.3 Smoothening Administrative Processes, Reducing Costs

AI has the potential for automation and optimization of administrative tasks; therein lies the key to increased operational efficiency, which reduces healthcare costs. It enables healthcare organizations to be more focused with their resources in delivering high-quality care for patients.

Routine Tasks Automation AI can automate time-consuming administrative tasks in areas such as scheduling, billing, and management of patient records. Artificial intelligence eases the burden on healthcare staff by freeing up highly valued time and resources to be redirected toward patients.

Efficient Allocation of Resources By aiding decision-making, analytics infused with AI can help healthcare providers optimize resource allocation, so that all patients may get attended to with adequate staffing and equipping. Train predictive models on historical trends to project admissions and demands for resources, which will guide and manage plans for better service delivery.

Fraud Detection and Risk Management Artificial intelligence can look for patterns in billing and claims data to identify fraudulent activities and consequently cut the losses in finances. Other than that, AI models can analyse risk factors, recognizing possible areas of concern and working towards managing risks for healthcare organizations.

It Brings About Cost Reduction Through Improved Efficiency Artificial intelligence optimizes operations and reduces the chances of errors, thereby contributing to cost savings in healthcare. The improved diagnostic accuracy and customized treatment plans will mean that resources are utilized more effectively and many such unnecessary procedures that inflate healthcare costs are avoided.

1.4 Challenges of AI in Healthcare

While AI does indeed offer significant hope for changing health care, actual implementation is also joined by some core difficulties. Development and deployment of AI in the health context involve surmounting a host of technical challenges, achieving interoperability with a legacy of diverse systems, and managing intrinsic complexity in health care data. This section examines some of the important challenges and their consequences on the health industry.

1.4.1 Technical Challenges in Developing and Implementing AI Systems

Several technical challenges shall be addressed in the development and implementation of AI systems in healthcare to make them effective and reliable.

Algorithm Complexity and Model Training Most advanced AI algorithms involve deep architectures, along with a large amount of training data, to obtain high accuracy and generalization, which can be computationally expensive to develop and require expertise in AI and machine learning. Further, training can be prohibitively time- and resource-consuming in an organization within the health care domain, with minimal access to state-of-the-art computational infrastructure.

Data Quality and Availability AI is very dependent on the quality of their training and validation data. Medical data may be missing, inconsistent, or wrong. This would bring down AI models' performance. Thus, ensuring high data quality and its availability is, therefore, the most critical challenge, as AI requires a large diverse dataset for learning purposes and to make accurate predictions. Moreover, adequate labelled data for training supervised learning tasks can be hard to get, especially in specialized medical domains.

Bias and Fairness AI models may sometimes even learn biased training data, which goes on to give biased predictions and outcomes. In healthcare, biased AI systems lead to unequal treatment of patients and different healthcare service delivery. No bias and fairness in AI means careful preprocessing of the data, transparency of algorithms, and continuous monitoring for early detection and reducing biased behaviour.

Explainability and Transparency Most AI models, more so the deep learning models, are often called "black box" due to the lack of interpretability. For example, in health, there is a reported lack of explanation for AI-driven decisions that poses challenges for clinicians who need to understand the rationale behind recommendations. Equipping AI systems with explainable and transparent outputs will gain trust and facilitate informed decision-making.

1.4.2 Interoperability Issues with Existing Healthcare Systems

One of the major challenges for integrating AI systems into existing healthcare infrastructure is interoperability. Most often, great dependence is upon various systems and platforms; all of them should work in integration for the successful implementation of AI.

Fragmented Healthcare Systems Most of the healthcare systems are fragmented, and this is the case in many departments with different software and data formats in use. This lack of standardization has retarded the integration of AI systems; such systems require homogeneous and interoperable data sources to work effectively. Since interoperability requires the aligning of AI technologies with previously existing systems and standards, it can turn out to be very intricate and involves a lot of resources.

Data Silos Health organizations traditionally hold data in isolated silos, leading to the issue of an inability to access a complete data set for AI systems to use. Such silos are created either because of proprietary software, legacy systems, or regulatory restrictions. Working across these silos involves developing data-sharing protocols and ensuring that AI systems can get the information they need to yield useful results.

EHR Integration While some of the most critical sources for patient information, there are many challenges associated with the integration of AI systems into EHR platforms due to incompatibility problems and differing standards for data. The seamless integration of these AI tools with the EHR is key to delivering actionable insights at the point of care.

Standard and Regulatory Compliance AI systems should make use of the standards and regulations for the health industries, such as HL7 and FHIR, to interoperate with existing healthcare infrastructure. Compliance with these standards is required for interoperability to be realized but can be complex due to the complexity and variability of the healthcare environments.

1.4.3 Managing the Complexity of Healthcare Data

The complexity of healthcare data is usually epitomized by its volume, variety, and velocity. The complexities of the data, very often, pose a range of challenges that any AI system should be able to handle.

Volume of Data Healthcare generates huge volumes of data arising from many sources, such as medical records, imaging studies, and wearable devices. AI systems have to be empowered to process this amount of data to produce meaningful insights. Large volumes of data need efficient mechanisms of storage, processing, and retrieval, besides robust algorithms with the capacity for high-dimensional data.

Variety in Data Type This data can be structured data, such as lab results, unstructured data, such as clinical notes, and even multivariate data, like images and videos. Consequently, AI models are burdened with processing multi-modal data and fusing the results in producing a coherent view about overall patient health. That's why working with multi-modal data would be kind of complex, especially while incorporating advanced NLP and computer vision techniques during model development.

Information Security and Privacy Healthcare data is very sensitive and has to be protected to hold the privacy of patients' information and be in compliance with regulations such as HIPAA and GDPR. AI systems have to take sufficient measures to protect healthcare data against unauthorized access and breaches. Last but not least, maintaining data privacy while ensuring data utility for the training and evaluation of AI models is another complex challenge, and techniques include data anonymization and federated learning.

Dynamic and Evolving Data All healthcare data is dynamic and constantly evolving in nature, reflecting changes in patients' health and the treatment protocol.

Accordingly, AI systems will have to be versatile and learn from new data continuously to stay relevant and accurate. One of the important challenges in healthcare AI currently is developing models capable of updating and becoming more accurate over time without requiring complete retraining (Fig. 1.2).

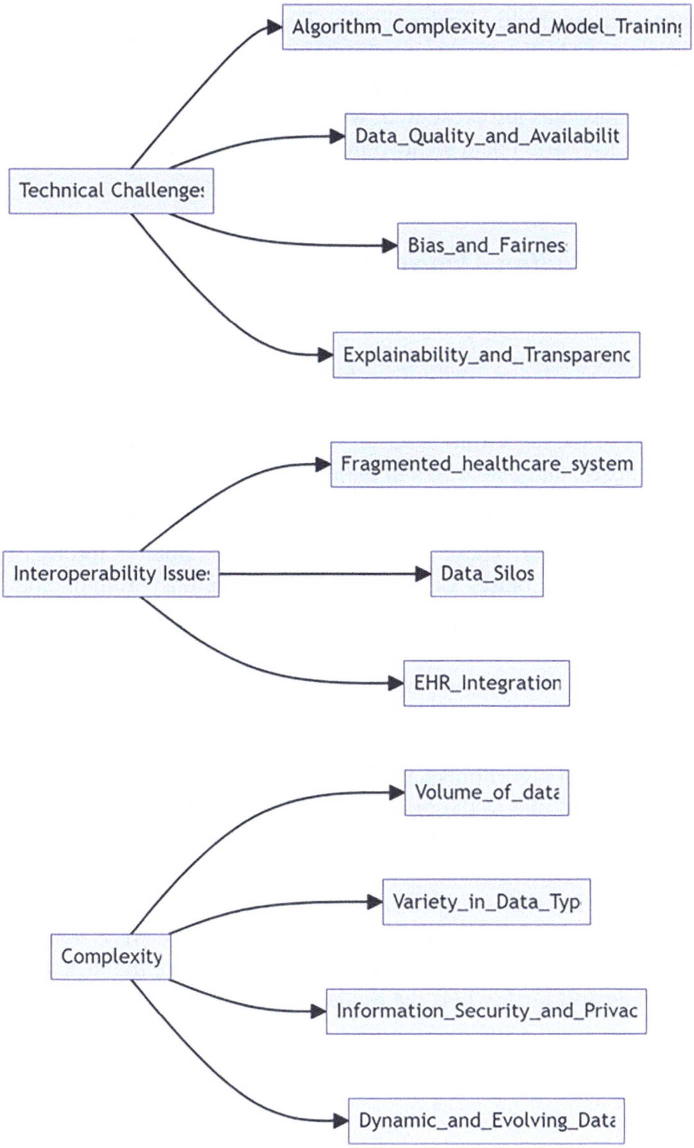

Fig. 1.2 Challenges of AI in Healthcare

1.5 Bias and Fairness in AI Algorithms

Ensuring fairness and mitigating the bias in algorithms are key in the mainstreaming of artificial intelligence into the healthcare delivery system. AI algorithms may support important improvements in health outcomes, but at the same time, they carry the risk of being implemented in ways that differentiate or even exacerbate pre-existing disparities in health. Understanding bias in AI models is a key step toward the goal of attaining health equity in minimizing disparities around patient care. In general, within this section, the sources and effects of the algorithmic bias and the ways to reduce this bias are presented, where special attention is paid to the influence exerted by the varied data set toward promoting fairness.

1.5.1 Understanding Algorithm Bias and Its Inducing Effect on Healthcare Outcomes

Algorithmic bias is a latent form of systemic and unfair discrimination in the AI models arising due to the heuristic data on which they are trained, or it could be an inherent feature of the algorithm itself. In healthcare, bias can lead to unequal treatment, misdiagnoses, and disparities in patient outcomes.

Sources of Algorithmic Bias

Training on Biased Data: These models learn their parameters through past data, which may contain biases or otherwise, perturbations brought about by the imbalances in the health care delivery system. If the data are skewed with biases, an AI model designed on such data will inherit these biases. A dataset that consists mostly of one particular demographic group will dampen the performance of an AI model on underrepresented groups, creating a prediction that is biased with a corresponding outcome.

Algorithm Design: AI algorithms have been designed and architected, which means they can be biased due to the priority set on some features or attributes against others. Poor feature selection or weighting naturally leads to biased models that are favorable to certain groups of people.

Feedback Loops: AI systems may create feedback loops where biased outcomes can eventually reinforce existing biases. For example, if an AI system continually underestimates some condition within a minority group, the lack of data about the treatments will further bias the model's predictions.

1.5.2 *Impact on Health Care*

Unequal Treatment Bias in AI may lead to unequal access to treatments and health care resources being accorded to different populations. An example would be the underestimation of the risk for female patients to have heart disease; therefore, fewer diagnostic tests are run and there is less intensive intervention for females, including minority females, and hence an increase in disparities in health.

Misdiagnoses and Errors This cause of concern in the case of AI-model-related bias would lead to misdiagnoses, particularly in the case of underrepresented groups. Such eventualities could bring in delayed or mismatched treatment on the patient with harmful effects on the health of the patient.

Health Disparities Algorithmic bias can further magnify existing health disparities by reinforcing unequal delivery of health care. For ensuring fairness in AI systems for the promotion of health equity and improvement of health outcomes for all patients.

1.5.3 *Bias Reduction Strategies in AI Model*

To achieve fairness and equality in AI systems, healthcare will need to adopt the following strategies—detection and mitigation of bias in AI models:

Bias Detected and Evaluated
Regular Audits and Testing: AI models must be audited and tested periodically for bias related to different demographic groups. This includes periodically reviewing the model's performance and identifying different predictions or outcomes. Methods, such as fairness metrics, could be used to quantifiably measure bias and review model fairness.

Transparency and Interpretability
A transparent and interpretable model for AI-based functions could reveal possible biases in the making of the model. Transparent models imply that the healthcare provider should be capable of following the reasonability behind AI-made decisions to catch pitfalls within the decision-making process that could reflect bias.

Algorithmic Interventions
Fairness Constraints. The design of the algorithm might introduce the constraint of fairness, which would act to temper the bias. Fairness-aware algorithms adjust performance to ensure that it is equal across groups—to reduce disparity in the outcomes.

Reweighting and Rebalancing It basically reweights the features with less influence. If features have different weights, for the balance of training data, the sum of instances across the minority cases' features is sampled without replacement. The balancing technique will ensure an appropriate representation of the racial or ethnic group during the model training process.

1.5.4 Collaborative Approaches

Interdisciplinary Collaboration: There is a need for collaboration between the data scientists, healthcare professionals, and ethicists to design an AI system that is transparent and fair, and therefore they will be in a better place to get a divergent perspective.

Stakeholder Engagement Engagement of stakeholders in the process of AI system development and evaluation, including patients and community representatives, is crucial for the detection of biases and to ensure the models meet community needs and values that might differ widely.

Role of Diverse Datasets for Fairness
Diverse and representative datasets are the base for any development of fair AI models that will lead to fair health outcomes.

Importance of Diversity in Data
Allow for More Comprehensive Representation of Diverse Data: In this way, capturing the heterogeneity of the patient population using diverse datasets would make the AI models generalizable across different demographic groups. High levels of comprehensive representation would reduce potential risks of bias, thereby leading to better model performance for all patients.
Fairness: Diversity within the training-data set of model development in AI implementation in healthcare organizations will contribute to the fairness of AI systems during patient treatment and sourcing care services. Diverse data helps AI systems recognize and address the unique needs of underrepresented groups.

1.5.5 Challenges and Considerations

Collection and Curation of Data Data should be collected with diversity in its nature, and the demographic factors like age, gender, race, ethnicity, and socioeconomic status need to be considered. Quality of data and completeness will be of prime concern to completely allow the model to get appropriately trained and evaluated.

Data Balancing Even with diverse datasets, imbalances may occur when some groups are underrepresented or overrepresented. Techniques allowing oversampling, undersampling, and creating synthetic data address these imbalances and hence promote fairness.

Privacy and Ethical Concerns The heterogeneous datasets should comply with the ethical standards and regulations regarding the privacy of data. In protecting the rights of patients and their trust, patient consent and data anonymization must be observed.

1.6 Ethical Considerations in AI Healthcare

Although the integration of artificial intelligence into health systems shows enormous potential for improving patient outcomes, enhancing medical research, and smoothening operations, the adoption of AI technologies also puts forward significant ethical concerns that have to be duly addressed to ensure that patients' rights are respected and ethical precepts upheld. This section considers some of the pressing ethical considerations around artificial intelligence in health, with regard to the balance between innovation and protection of the rights of patients, informed consent and transparency, and the kinds of ethical pitfalls that may be opened up by these technologies.

1.6.1 Balancing Innovation with Patient Rights and Ethical Principles

While AI continues to drive innovation in healthcare, technological development must be balanced against the protection of patient rights and ethical principles to ensure that AI systems are developed responsibly.

Respect for Autonomy

Patient-Centered Care: AI systems should protect the autonomy of patients through active support in informed decision-making and respect for preferences. Patients shall be empowered to make decisions in their choices regarding healthcare decisions, consonant with their values and beliefs.

Shared Decision-Making: AI technologies shall facilitate shared decision-making between patients and healthcare providers. AI systems can facilitate this collaboration by making relevant and appropriate information available in order for patients to actively engage in care.

Beneficence and Non-Maleficence

Maximize the Benefits: AI systems should aim to realize benefits for the patients by improving diagnostic accuracy, treatment effectiveness, and health outcomes in general. Ensuring that AI technologies can actually provide some benefits is an ethical imperative.

Harm Reduction: Such risks and harms that an AI system might pose need to be carefully evaluated and minimized, such as algorithm bias, violation of data security, and mistakes in AI-driven recommendations that may pose a negative impact on health.

Justice and Fairness

Fair access: It should be done by AI technologies in health care, making provision for fair access to the available health resources and ensuring that each patient gets appropriate care, no matter their backgrounds or socio-economic status. Addressing health disparities in the delivery of health care is thus of great importance so that the principle of justice can be upheld.

Resource Allocation: AI systems can contribute to the distribution of scarce health care resources by determining the needs of the patient and optimizing treatment plans. Conversely, transparency in resource allocation decisions is called for and should be strictly based on ethical principles.

1.6.2 Informed Consent and Transparency of AI-Driven Decisions

Ethics in artificial intelligence systems simply means that a patient shall have proper information with respect to how AI technologies are going to affect his or her healthcare, and such decisions taken are completely clear and understandable by him or her. Informed Consent:

Patient Awareness: Patients should be made aware of the use of AI technologies in their care, including descriptions of AI system functions, data they will use, and likely impacts on diagnosis and treatment. Informed consent is meaningful only when there is clear communication.

Voluntary participation: The patient should be given the opportunity to either elect or refuse AI-driven intervention without being coerced. Participation can be treated as purely voluntary and based on a good understanding of AI technologies in the interest of patient autonomy and ethical decision-making.

Transparency of AI Systems

Explainability and Interpretability: AI systems shall be in a position to provide an explanation for their decisions and recommendations, thus allowing the patients and health providers to understand what lies beneath AI-driven outcomes. Explainability will foster the development of trust and confidence in AI technologies.

Disclosure of Limitations: Patients and health professionals should be told about the limitations and uncertainties of the models. Understanding the limitations of AI capabilities avoids raising false expectations about its appropriate use.

Communication and Engagement

Patient Engagement: Engaging patients in the use of AI technologies in the delivery of health care can increase transparency and lead to greater collaboration. Patient feedback may reveal insights into ethical implications associated with AI systems and inform their development and deployment.

1.6.3 Resolving Ethical Dilemmas Within AI Applications

Applications of AI in Health Care can give rise to complex ethical dilemmas that call for scrupulous consideration and thought-out resolution for ensuring the maintenance of ethical practices.

Data Privacy and Confidentiality One of the key ethical duties to avoid unauthorized access and breaches would be to ensure robust measures of protection of the patient's data in AI systems that require vast amounts of sensitive patient data.

Anonymization and De-identification Guaranteeing the privacy of the patient due to techniques such as anonymization and de-identification of data protects the patients, yet still keeps the data useful for training and testing AI models.

Bias and Discrimination

Identification and Mitigation of Bias: The development of AI systems in various fields has been supposed to address bias in order to prevent discriminatory practices in healthcare delivery. Fairness-aware algorithms are to be implemented in the design of models for ethical AI using different datasets that bring down bias and advance justice.

Monitoring and Accountability: There is a need to implement monitoring and accountability mechanisms to identify and deal with the biases of AI systems. Therefore, healthcare institutions should ensure the identification of possible biases and take remedial measures for the same.

Algorithmic Accountability

Outcome Responsibility: There is a decline in accountability for AI-driven decisions with cases of errors or adverse outcomes. It is very critical from an ethical dimension that AI systems enhance the human element and not supplant it.

Ethical Oversight: AI machines and their systems must be under ethical scrutiny and supervision, so that their development and deployment shall align with ethical precepts. It can be presided and overseen by independent review boards and ethics committees over responsible AI practices.

Balancing Innovation with Regulation

Regulatory Compliance: AI systems should be designed in a manner that allows them to respect existing regulations and standards for their safe and ethical application. Striking a balance between innovation and regulation, the development of responsible AI will help to retain public trust.

Ethical Innovation: The promotion of ethical innovation entails the internalization of ethical considerations at the very point of designing and developing AI systems. Ethical frameworks and guidelines could help guide AI innovation so as to ensure that new technologies safeguard the rights and wellbeing of patients.

Successful implementation of AI in healthcare requires directly embedding ethical considerations into its operations. Innovations can be balanced against patient rights and ethical principles, informed consent, transparency, and management of ethical dilemmas to ensure the development of AI systems that are responsible, guaranteeing health organizations deliver care equitably. Moving forward with AI development, continued effort in the face of such ethical challenges holds the key to unlocking the full potential of AI in improving patient outcomes and changing health care delivery.

1.7 Best Practices for Ensuring Privacy and Security

If artificial intelligence is integrated into health systems, stringent measures of privacy and security will have to be observed in order to maintain sensitive patient data safely; otherwise, faith in AI technologies may fade out. This is most important with the rise in volume and variety of healthcare data processing through AI systems. Best Practices to Protect Privacy and Security in AI-driven Healthcare This subsection outlines best practices in data protection within the context of AI health care, i.e., adopting adequate measures on data protection, designing models that protect privacy, and involving stakeholders in discussions on privacy.

1.7.1 Use of Adequate Measures for Robust Data Protection

An adequate level of data protection would guarantee that a patient's personal information would not be transferred or disclosed to unauthorized parties or individuals access to information related to one's health would not be allowed to be accessed by persons who are not authorized. Strong security practices ensure the terms confidentiality, integrity, and availability are maintained for data within the AI system.

Data Encryption

At Rest and in Transit: All healthcare data should either be stored or sent using industry-standard encryption algorithms. The data at rest will be encrypted to safeguard against any unauthorized access to the stored information; similarly, while being sent across a network, the data will be encrypted in transit.

End-to-End Encryption: This ensures that the health information is well protected right from its point of collection to the final destination, protecting it from probable interception and tampering.

Access and Authentication Controls

RBAC (Role-Based Access Control): It ensures in AI systems that access to certain data and functionalities is only available to duly authorized people. As per roles and responsibilities, users should have access permissions for restricting the exposure of sensitive data.

MFA (Multi-Factor Authentication): This involves more than one factor for authentication, making it more secure by authenticated checks and verification from the user's identity through multiple authentication factors like passwords, biometrics, or one-time codes.

Data Anonymization and De-identification

Anonymization Techniques: Anonymizing data means removing or obscuring personally identifiable information so that a patient's information is privacy-protected. This will be done by applying techniques such as data masking, aggregation, and generalization for anonymizing sensitive information, while keeping data utility intact.

De-Identification Standards: Setting standards in place for the de-identification of data will ensure prevention from easy re-identification or tracing of data items back to patients. De-identified data is completely safe for use in training AI models or analysis without giving away any information about the patients.

Data Minimization and Retention

Data minimization principle: The data minimization principle suggests collecting only those data that are relevant for the purpose. The lesser the collection and storage, the lesser are the chances of a breach, providing greater protection for privacy.

Data Retention Policies: Clear data retention policies of an organization ensure that it retains data only until it is mandated to do so; once the time period is over, the data must be securely deleted or archived.

Monitoring and Incident Response

Continuous Monitoring: Continuous monitoring in AI systems of data access seeks to detect all forms of suspicious activities in real time, and hence, any form of possible security breach. The monitoring tools will be able to identify anomalies and alert security teams for direct action.

Incident Response Plan: An in-depth incident response plan outlining procedures to be taken when a data breach or a security incident occurs. The plan has to be tested and updated often for the organization to properly deal with any security threats if and when they occur.

1.7.2 Design of Privacy-Preserving AI Models

The design of AI models that respect the privacy in the dataset while ensuring model's performance and utility includes multiple methodologies.

Federated Learning The method of decentralized model training is known as federated learning in which the AI model is trained on many decentralized devices/servers while data is kept on local devices without centralizing it. By doing so, this methodology preserves privacy by limiting the dynamics of data and consequently related risks of breaches.

Aggregation of Model Updates Federated learning shares model updates from the device and does not share raw data to ensure that sensitive information is not exposed or transmitted.

Differential Privacy

Privacy-Preserving Mechanisms: Differential privacy carries out perturbation, either on the data or model outputs, so created AI models will not be able to make any inference about specific pieces of information related to the individual patients; at the same time, these are statistically accurate.

Balancing Privacy and Utility: The amount of noise added to the data should be related to the utility sought in the model being learned. Hence, careful tuning of this amount is necessary to retain privacy while guaranteeing a reasonable model performance. Secure multi-party computation:

Collaborative data processing: SMPC can execute a computation that involves multiple parties on their private data items without exposing their respective inputs to one another. Granger techniques allow privacy-preserving data analysis and model training across organizations.

Confidentiality in Data: It ensures that private and sensitive data is concealed throughout the process of its computation, restricting any unauthorized access and thus protecting the privacy of the patients.

Homomorphic Encryption

Encrypted data processing: Homomorphic encryption allows the operations of a computation to be done on the data in its encrypted form. In this idea, it allows the training and inference of artificial intelligence models with private health data in privacy-preserving ways.

Secure data: Because homomorphic encryption includes data processing in an encrypted state, patient data is secured and remains private even when being used in complicated computations.

1.7.3 Engaging Stakeholders in Privacy Discussions and Decision-Making

Stakeholders need to be involved in the privacy-related discourse and decision-making processes, to instil trust, allay their various concerns, and have AI systems aligned with ethical and privacy standards.

Stakeholder Engagement

Engagement of Patients: Engaging patients within the privacy discourse ensures that AI systems are designed and implemented considering their perspectives, preferences, and concerns. It builds trust and transparency into AI-driven health care by engaging patients.

Engaging healthcare professionals in privacy decision-making for the adoption of AI systems will ensure such a process aligns with the clinical workflow and meets practitioners' needs. Healthcare professionals can provide very valuable insights into ethical and practical implications of AI technologies.

Privacy Impact Assessments

Risk Assessment: PIAs estimate probable privacy risks related to AI systems and define the measures to reduce these risks. PIAs provide for the fact that privacy considerations are taken into account while designing and fielding AI technologies.

Involving stakeholders in PIAs ensures diversified perspectives that would guide in jointly addressing privacy risks with the stakeholders. Privacy strategies and effectiveness in conducting PIAs may benefit from input by stakeholders.

Clear and Transparent Communication

Clear Privacy Policies: Clear and readily available privacy policies empower patients and all stakeholders so that they fully comprehend how AI systems use and protect their data. This requires clear and transparent communication to imbue trust and reliance on AI technologies.

Continuing Dialogue: Continuous dialogue among stakeholders regarding privacy practices and the updating process forms a guarantee that AI continues to be aligned with any changing privacy standards and expectations. Continuous communication fosters collaboration and accountability.

Aggregation of privacy and security in healthcare AI applications engulfs the incorporation of strong data protection measures and the design of privacy-preserving models of AI, thereby engaging its stakeholders in discussions and decisions about privacy. Best practices and respect for patients' privacy will help healthcare organizations gain trust in AI technologies and protect sensitive data. Ethics and responsible care will be within reach. As AI is on the way to dramatically change health care, continued efforts to meet challenges related to privacy and security will be required if public trust is to be maintained and successful integration of AI into health care systems ensured.

1.8 Conclusion

Artificial intelligence applied to healthcare has the potential to bring fundamental changes, offering several advantages in terms of diagnosis accuracy, treatment management, and operational efficiency. At the same time, challenges exist in the adoption of AI technologies, including technical challenges on many levels, interoperability, algorithm bias, and the ethical complexities of privacy and patient consent. The following are challenges that healthcare systems are yet to resolve if AI is to live up to its potential: robust measures of data protection, designs for privacy-preserving AI models, and transparency and collaboration among all stakeholders. Eventually, when AI will further develop in the future, ethical conduct and equal rights are indispensable for exploiting AI's potential in order to ensure AI-driven innovation has a positive effect on patient care and that the evolution of health sciences takes place in a responsible way.

References

1. S. Hensel, B. Jagusch and T. Lux, "Introduction of Artificial Intelligence in Healthcare Lectures: An Evaluation," 2023 20th ACS/IEEE International Conference on Computer Systems and Applications (AICCSA), Giza, Egypt, 2023, pp. 1–5, https://doi.org/10.1109/AICCSA59173.2023.10479324.
2. R. Nidhya; Manish Kumar; R. Maheswar; D. Pavithra, "Security and Privacy Issues in Smart Healthcare System Using Internet of Things," in IoT-enabled Smart Healthcare Systems, Services and Applications, Wiley, 2022, pp. 63–85, https://doi.org/10.1002/9781119816829.ch4.
3. P. Wang and H. Zare, "A Case Study of Privacy Protection Challenges and Risks in AI-Enabled Healthcare App," 2023 IEEE Conference on Artificial Intelligence (CAI), Santa Clara, CA, USA, 2023, pp. 296–297, https://doi.org/10.1109/CAI54212.2023.00132.
4. Romagnoli, A., Ferrara, F., Langella, R. et al. Healthcare Systems and Artificial Intelligence: Focus on Challenges and the International Regulatory Framework. Pharm Res 41, 721–730 (2024). https://doi.org/10.1007/s11095-024-03685-3
5. Ueda, D., Kakinuma, T., Fujita, S. et al. Fairness of artificial intelligence in healthcare: review and recommendations. Jpn J Radiol 42, 3–15 (2024). https://doi.org/10.1007/s11604-023-01474-3
6. Herzog, N.J., Celik, D., Sulaiman, R.B. (2024). Artificial Intelligence in Healthcare and Medical Records Security. In: Jahankhani, H., Bowen, G., Sharif, M.S., Hussien, O. (eds) Cybersecurity and Artificial Intelligence. Advanced Sciences and Technologies for Security Applications. Springer, Cham. https://doi.org/10.1007/978-3-031-52272-7_2

Chapter 2
Sensor Based IOT Enabled Healthcare Systems and Role of AI and Security

Contents

Abstract This review critically analyses the transforming terrain of sensor-based IoT-enabled healthcare systems and their connected aspects with an eye toward the complex interaction between components, the fusion of IoT and healthcare, and the vital junction between artificial intelligence (AI) and security. By means of analysis of the components of wearable devices, medical instruments, data transmission techniques, cloud platforms, and user interfaces in sensor-based healthcare systems, we may better understand their combined relevance in supporting real-time health monitoring and customized therapies. Investigating IoT integration into healthcare emphasizes the perfect device connectivity and consequent continuous data streams that enable patients and enhance healthcare services. Emphasizing the critical relevance of security in IoT applications for healthcare, the review provides an in-depth study of encryption mechanisms, authentication protocols, access restrictions, device integrity checks, and safe communication protocols, stressing their indispensable role in preserving the confidentiality and integrity of private health data. Furthermore, the study focuses on how artificial intelligence impacts healthcare results by isolating its contributions in customized medicine, predictive modelling, and data analytics. A thorough examination of the existing status and problems, considering future paths of sensor-based IoT-enabled healthcare systems, contrib-

S. Gupta et al., *Artificial Intelligence-Enabled Security for Healthcare Systems*,
https://doi.org/10.1007/978-3-031-82810-2_2

utes to a fundamental grasp of the complex interplay between sensors, IoT, artificial intelligence, and security, thus directing the creation of intelligent and safe healthcare ecosystems.

Keywords IoT Healthcare · Healthcare Security · Artificial Intelligence · IoT Sensor

2.1 Introduction

Artificial intelligence (AI) and the Internet of Things (IoT), technological development has drastically changed the course of healthcare. Sensor-based IoT-enabled healthcare systems have evolved from better features in data collection, processing, and patient monitoring. Comprising wearable gadgets, environmental sensors, and robust diagnostic tools—which span a spectrum—these systems—which span a spectrum—are transforming healthcare delivery by delivering real-time, continuous monitoring and individualized therapy.

Still, the way these technologies are integrated raises major security concerns that have to be addressed if we are to protect patient data and ensure the authenticity and dependability of healthcare systems. This introduction first summarizes the consecutive expansion of artificial intelligence (AI), sensor-based Internet of Things (IoT) healthcare systems, and changing security emphasis (Fig. 2.1).

Originally starting in healthcare in the 1960s, IoT first experimented with online health monitoring and telemedicine. These early developments showed that medical

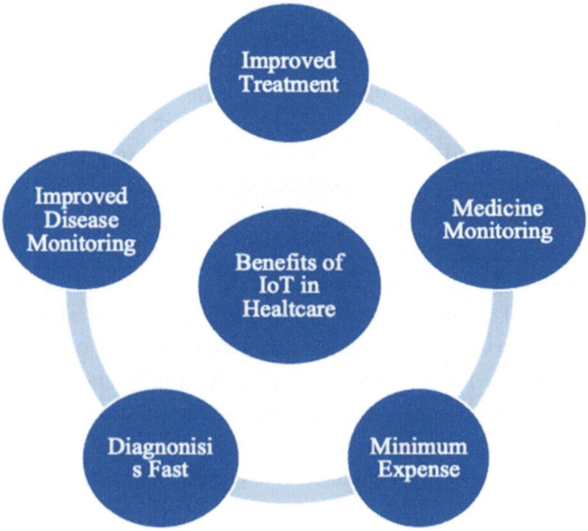

Fig. 2.1 Advantages of IoT-dependent health care

treatments could be provided at a distance, therefore laying the groundwork for modern telehealth applications. NASA's creative study of pilot health in space found that telemedicine was not only practical but also really important [2].

The route for eventual technological advancements in the medical profession was opened by these early efforts at online monitoring. Smart technology was a major breakthrough for sensor-based healthcare systems when it first surfaced in the 1980s. Among the first devices available were simple fitness trackers and heart rate monitors. These provide people and doctors with new ways to handle medical records. These novel ideas were very essential in allowing ever more advanced personal technology to manifest in the coming decades [3].

Kevin Ashton first used the phrase "Internet of Things" in 1999 to mark the start of a new age of linked devices defining our lives. People started quickly using this idea in many sectors, including medicine. In the 1990s and early 2000s, IoT technologies were added to medical devices like networked pacemakers and RFID-tag enabled stocking systems. Early IoT applications showed how improved monitoring and asset management may assist in improving healthcare [4].

In the 2010s, many more people started using smart health technology. When they first launched in 2009 and 2015, the Fitbit and Apple Watch transformed individuals' monitoring of their own health. Modern sensors added to these gadgets may track numerous physiological aspects, including activity level, heart rate, and sleep patterns. The data these gadgets gathered was helpful for individuals as well as for healthcare professionals, as it led to more proactive and tailored treatment [5].

Artificial intelligence and machine learning started to transform healthcare concurrently as they were added to IoT devices. Let us look at the massive amounts of data produced by IoT devices. Artificial intelligence algorithms enabled the simpler creation of personalized treatment plans and predictive analytics. For instance, IBM Watson Health's AI-powered diagnosis tools started helping doctors choose the best course of action and interpret complicated medical data [6]. The ability of healthcare systems to provide high-quality treatment depending on data mostly relies on the convergence of IoT and artificial intelligence (Fig. 2.2).

As the internet of things (IoT) extended across healthcare, security issues emerged. Healthcare data is so sensitive that cyber attackers find immense pleasure in it. IoT devices and the data they generate have to be safe and vital. Based on data breaches and intrusions on healthcare institutions under much public scrutiny, strong security measures are clearly needed. Therefore, building better encryption methods, blockchain technology for safe data management, and whole cybersecurity systems became quite important. These steps ensure that IoT healthcare systems run as they should, preserve patient data, and help to maintain confidence [7]. Sensor-based IoT-enabled healthcare systems are still developing today as artificial intelligence, hacking, and sensor technology are always advancing. The COVID-19 outbreak accelerated the use of telemedicine and remote tracking technologies, thereby proving the need for IoT in handling public health emergencies. For predictive analytics, blockchain use to provide data security, and 5G network rollout to satisfy the growing data needs of IoT healthcare systems going forward, people might be excited about ever more complex AI algorithms. Examining the history of

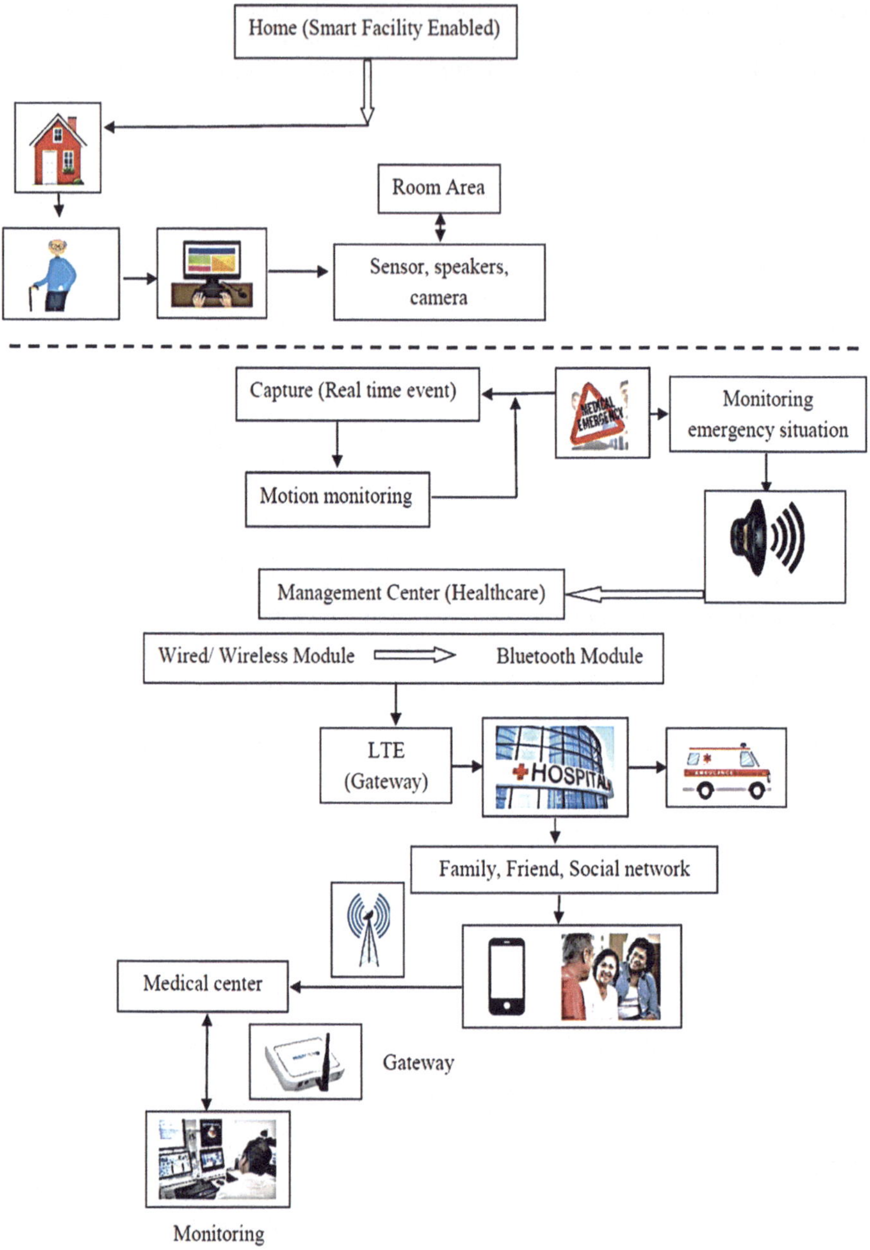

Fig. 2.2 IoT framework for healthcare systems [1]

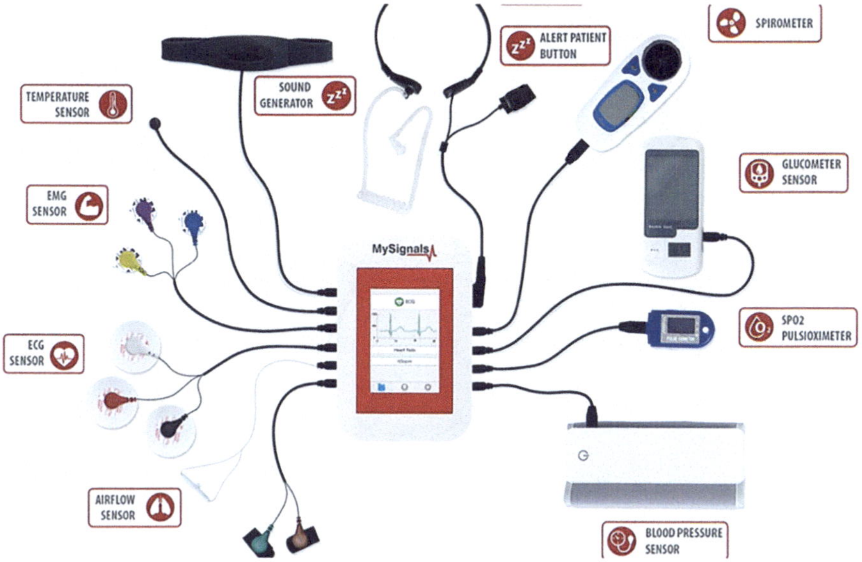

Fig. 2.3 Types of sensors in medical devices [9]

sensor-based IoT-enabled healthcare systems reveals quite interesting patterns, from the first attempts at remote tracking to the most advanced AI-driven solutions [8]. Combining IoT with artificial intelligence enables healthcare companies to provide targeted and preventative therapy significantly more simply. But the security problems surrounding it suggest that constant maintenance of private health data to ensure system operation depends on new ideas and determined measures. The path of healthcare will be shaped by how quickly and successfully these game-changing technologies are developed and implemented.

2.2 Components of Sensor-Based Healthcare Systems

sensor-based healthcare systems track, evaluate, and control patient health using these pieces. Among these elements are enhanced diagnosis tools, sensors for the surroundings, and wearable technology. Every one of these elements is very vital for IoT-enabled healthcare systems to operate as they should (Fig. 2.3).

Wearable Devices

Wearable gadgets are at the cutting edge of sensor-based healthcare systems because they can track physiological factors all the time. These gadgets have sensors that keep track of things like heart rate, blood pressure, glucose levels, and physical exercise. They include smartwatches, fitness trackers, and medical-grade wearables. As an example, the Apple Watch and Fitbit have become very popular ways to track

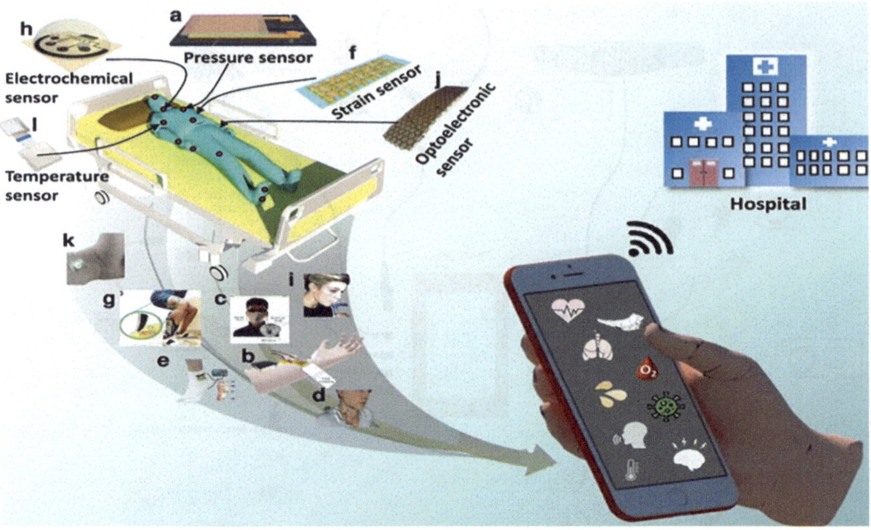

Fig. 2.4 IoT and sensor-based development for healthcare system [10]

and share important health information between users and healthcare professionals [5] (Fig. 2.4).

Wearable gadgets may currently help with customised healthcare measures and offer you further information about your health. Usually, these gadgets have numerous sensors—such as accelerometers, gyroscopes, and photo platysma grams (PPG)—to offer total health tracking. These wearables gather data that can be sent to doctors so they might review it in real time and offer fast medical solutions. This will make the healthcare system less busy and improve patient outcomes [11].

2.2.1 *Environmental Sensors*

Environmental devices provide a further crucial function in sensor-based healthcare systems.

Temperature, humidity, air quality, and light levels are among the factors these sensors track that could compromise a patient's health. Those who suffer from allergies or asthma should particularly pay great attention to their surroundings, as factors in such circumstances may worsen their symptoms. By continuously collecting data on the surroundings, these monitors can notify patients and medical staff about any threats, therefore facilitating prompt responses [12].

Advanced environmental sensors used in hospitals, residences, and other healthcare facilities guarantee that patients are in the best possible condition for treatment.

For instance, air quality sensors may find pollutants and allergens, which would enable one to control respiratory problems knowing this. Temperature and humidity sensors help to maintain settings appropriate for those with long-term disorders, therefore lowering the risk of issues and improving the overall standard of health care [13].

2.2.2 *Diagnostic Tools*

IoT-enabled diagnostic kits that can be linked to the internet of things (IoT) mark an important development in the way medical tests are executed. Among these tools are blood pressure cuffs, smart glucometers, and electrocardiogram (ECG) monitors. They may test and let doctors know the results right away. Since scans are readily incorporated into IoT systems, tests may be carried out rapidly and precisely; healthcare providers may also use real-time data to drive smart decisions [14].

By means of diagnostics, smart diagnostic devices using IoT technology offer remote tracking and diagnosis, therefore lowering the necessary hospital visits. For diabetics, smart glucometers help them to continuously monitor their blood sugar levels, therefore enhancing their control of them and generating more tailored treatment plans. Similarly, ECG monitoring enables early treatment and better patient outcomes by letting doctors know about likely cardiac problems [15].

2.2.3 *Data Integration and Analysis Platforms*

Wearable tech, outdoor sensors, and diagnostic tools create a lot of data, which means that strong systems are needed to combine and analyse that data. These systems compile, retain, and examine data to provide you with useful insights. Predictive analytics and tailored health recommendations are made feasible by the increasing use of artificial intelligence and machine learning techniques in handling this data [16, 17].

Healthcare providers can get complete and up-to-date integrated information about their patients. This improves the level of care and guarantees better treatment quality. These systems help doctors better know a patient's status by combining information from several sensors and devices. From this, follow more correct treatment plans and more accurate diagnoses. Furthermore, enabling us to foresee future occurrences and hence prevent bad health events as well as improve long-term health outcomes, AI-powered analytics can also spot trends and patterns in health data [17].

2.2.4 *Communication Networks*

IoT-enabled healthcare systems must have robust information networks to run. These systems enable medical personnel, sensors, and equipment to easily communicate and receive data. High-speed, low latency links—like those offered by 5G and other developing communication technologies [18]—define real-time health tracking and intervention. Wearable technologies and sensors allow strong communication networks to rapidly and safely transmit data to medical experts. This real-time data transmission helps doctors monitor patients continuously and administer rapid therapies, thereby improving the overall standard of healthcare. Sensor-based healthcare systems will be able to perform better when IoT technology keeps developing and more advanced communication networks are built [19].

2.3 Internet of Things (IoT) and Healthcare: Coordination and Technological Progress

In healthcare, the Internet of Things (IoT) has changed everything by providing new ways to improve patient care, make processes run more smoothly, and lead to better results. Several technologies and apps work together as IoT is used in healthcare to build a connected health environment. Emphasizing numerous significant technologies and their uses, this part discusses IoT's relevance in healthcare.

2.3.1 *How IoT and Healthcare Are Related*

In the context of healthcare, IoT refers to the network of connected devices and sensors compiling, sending, and analysing health data. All of which are fairly important for controlling chronic diseases, guaranteeing patients receive better treatment, and maximizing healthcare resources. These technologies offer continuous tracking, real-time data collection, and remote care. In healthcare, IoT devices include medical tools, smart home devices, and monitors that can be worn. All of these things work together to make a full healthcare network (Fig. 2.5).

The Internet of Things (IoT) is being used more and more in healthcare because of the need for more efficient care, the rise in chronic diseases, and improvements in sensor technology and data analytics. IoT finds use in many various fields, including healthcare, where it may be used to monitor patients from distance and provide telemedicine, in addition to build smart hospitals and perform predictive maintenance on medical equipment. Table 2.1 shows below the technology, its function and application.

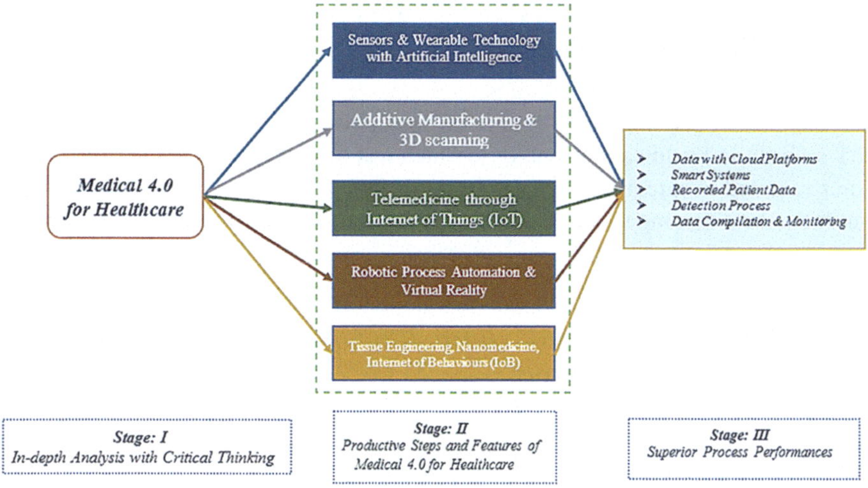

Fig. 2.5 Relational Diagram between IoT and healthcare [20]

Table 2.1 IoT enabled technology, function and application

Technology	Function	Applications
Wearable Sensors	Monitor physiological parameters and physical activity	Fitness tracking, chronic disease management, and post-operative monitoring
Environmental Sensors	Monitor ambient conditions that affect health	Air quality monitoring, temperature and humidity control, and smart home health management
Smart Diagnostic Tools	Conduct medical tests and transmit results to healthcare providers	monitoring, continuous glucose monitoring, ECG monitoring, and blood pressure monitoring
Telemedicine Platforms	Enable remote consultations and virtual care	Remote doctor visits, mental health counselling, and chronic disease management
AI and Machine Learning	AnalyzeAnalyse health data and provide predictive insights	Predictive analytics, personalized treatment plans, and early disease detection
Blockchain Technology	Ensure secure and transparent data management	Secure patient data exchange, electronic health records (EHRs), clinical trial management
5G Communication Networks	Provide high-speed, low-latency data transmission	telemedicine, andReal-time remote monitoring, telemedicine, augmented reality (AR) for surgery and training
Smart Hospital Systems	Automate and optimize hospital operations	Asset tracking, patient flow management, predictive maintenance of medical equipment

2.4 Security for IoT Used in Healthcare Systems: A Chronological Insight

The complexity and number of connected devices in medical contexts have changed IoT security in healthcare technology, which has helped to change the safety measures required to safeguard personal health information. This part shows, throughout time, the changing security measures used in IoT-enabled healthcare systems.

2.4.1 Early Developments: Basic Encryption and Access Controls

When IoT was first being used in healthcare in the late 1990s and early 2000s, security procedures were relatively straightforward. Two fundamental encryption methods—symmetric key encryption and access control—were applied to keep the data sent between devices safe. At first, the main focus was on ensuring only approved users could access private medical details. To do this, technologies like Secure Sockets Layer (SSL) were used to secure communication [21].

2.4.2 The Rise of More Advanced Encryption Protocols

As IoT devices multiplied in healthcare, more robust security measures became absolutely essential. Common standard practice in the 2010s emerged from Advanced Encryption Standard (AES) and Transport Layer Security (TLS) for advanced encryption protocols. These solutions provided robust encryption for data in transit and at rest from unauthorized access, therefore preserving patient information's confidentiality and security [22].

2.4.3 Introduction of Blockchain Technology (Mid-2010s)

Blockchain technology first found use in healthcare to improve data security and accuracy around middle of the 2010s. The independent and immutable log system of blockchain enables secure administration of electronic health records (EHRs) and other sensitive data. Blockchain technology has been shown to be a consistent tool for confirming validity and monitoring source of medical data [23]. It achieved this by making sure data could not be changed or deleted without being found.

2.4.4 *Development of AI-Driven Security Solutions (Late 2010s-Present)*

Around the end of the 2010s and beginning of the 2020s, AI and ML started to play a bigger part in IoT security. Using machine learning methods, artificial intelligence-powered security systems sought trends and anomalies in real time, safeguarding against cyberattacks before it started. These technologies allowed us to identify potential security flaws and unethical behaviour and provided a flexible and rapid means of safeguarding IoT settings in health care system.

2.4.5 *Implementation of Zero Trust Architecture (2020s)*

In the 2020s, Zero Trust Architecture (ZTA) was used because IoT platforms in healthcare were getting more complicated. Zero Trust approaches every device, user, and component of the network as always under authenticity and permission verification before it can access resources based on the idea of "never trust, always verify." This method reduced the likelihood of data theft by hackers, therefore giving IoT systems a full security framework suitable for their changing nature (National Institute of Standards and Technology [NIST], 2020) [25].

2.4.6 *Adoption of Quantum-Resistant Cryptography (Future Directions)*

Since quantum computing grows, it will make it harder for present encryption methods to work. Quantum based security is under development to protect IoT data from future hazards, like quantum computers. These complex security methods are meant to run inside quantum computer processing capacity. This will guarantee the confidentiality of medical data in the years after quantum computing [26] (Table 2.2).

2.5 Challenges and Limitations in Sensor-Based IoT Enabled Healthcare Systems

2.5.1 *Technological and Operational Challenges*

Interoperability Issues Integration of many IoT devices from different manufacturers sometimes results in compatibility issues, which limit data standardization and platform connectivity. Lack of interoperability can prevent perfect patient data sharing, therefore affecting the efficiency of healthcare services.

Table 2.2 Advancement of technology and their job

Period	Technological development	Description
1990s–2000s	Basic Encryption and Access Controls	Initial security measures use SSL and basic encryption to protect data transmission [21]
2010s	Advanced Encryption Protocols	Adoption of AES and TLS for robust data encryption [27]
Mid-2010s	Blockchain Technology	Implementation of blockchain for secure, immutable health data management [28]
Late 2010s-Present	AI-Driven Security Solutions	Use of AI and ML for real-time threat detection and adaptive security [24]
2020s	Zero Trust Architecture	Continuous authentication and authorization of devices and users [26]
Future Directions	Quantum-Resistant Cryptography	development of cryptographic algorithms to protect data against quantum computing threats [29]

Data Management and Storage The massive amount of data generated by Internet of Things devices needs robust data management and storage solutions. Ensuring that data is readily retrievable, reasonably stored, and compliant with healthcare regulations (like HIPAA) presents serious challenges.

Latency and Connectivity Low latency, fast speed Internet connections are prerequisites for real-time data tracking and processing. IoT healthcare solutions would not be as successful in places with limited internet access, which would cause slower data transfer and sporadic patient observation.

Device Reliability and Maintenance IoT devices used in healthcare should be trustworthy so that patients might be constantly monitored. If devices are to remain operational and protect patients, they must be frequently maintained, updated as needed, and tech problems fixed right away.

2.5.2 *Security and Privacy Challenges*

Cybersecurity Threats

IoT devices might come across cybersecurity risks such as hacking, data breaches, and virus attacks. It is always tough to keep patient information safe from individuals who shouldn't have access to it and make it indisputable that healthcare processes are authentic.

Data Privacy Concerns Privacy concerns surround the gathering and dissemination of private medical records. Maintaining patient confidence and respect for the law depends on patient data being protected, anonymized, and only shared with permitted staff.

Regulatory Compliance Ensuring regulatory compliance may be difficult as it entails, in many different nations and jurisdictions, varying and continually changing regulatory duties. Healthcare providers have to be sure their Internet of Things (IoT) systems satisfy data security laws like the General Data Protection Regulation (GDPR) in Europe and the Health Insurance Portability and Accountability Act (HIPAA) in United States.

Cost and Scalability Deployment of healthcare-related safe Internet of Things (IoT) requires a significant upfront investment. If related expenses seem excessively high, smaller healthcare providers may be discouraged from implementing, maintaining, and expanding IoT systems.

2.5.3 Future Directions and Emerging Solutions

Enhanced Interoperability Standards Work is underway to develop globally IoT device compatibility requirements for use in healthcare, hence improving interoperability guidelines. By streamlining procedures, these criteria will help ensure data exchange free from difficulties, system collaboration, and overall efficiency of healthcare services.

Advanced AI and Machine Learning IoT devices will be able to produce more accurate predictions as artificial intelligence and machine learning technologies keep improving. This will lead to further accurate diagnoses, more tailored treatment plans, and the prior discovery of health difficulties.

Quantum-Resistant Cryptography As quantum computing gets enhanced, it will be significant to generate quantum-resistant cryptographic methods to keep healthcare data safe from future computer risks. This will guarantee, over time, that IoT enabled healthcare systems stay safe and private.

Edge Computing Processing data closer to the source (at the network's edge) will lower delay when edge computing is used. IoT systems will therefore be more reliable, data processing in real time will be easier, and they will be less dependent on centralized cloud infrastructure.

Blockchain for Data Security Future maintenance of healthcare data safety will mostly rely on blockchain technology. Its consistent and unchangeable nature guarantees data integrity, thereby enabling secure data transfer across stakeholders, and helps to manage patient information by means of a strong, secure system.

Regulatory Framework Development Work is still under progress to bring uniformity of regulatory regimes all around. This will let medical experts follow rules more easily. Consistent standards and well-defined rules will help ease the moral and safe application of IoT technologies in healthcare.

Sensor-based IoT-enabled healthcare systems have an optimistic future ahead of them, as novel technologies possess to solve problems and make them better. Healthcare providers can ensure the secure, efficient, and effective utilization of IoT devices by implementing fresh innovations and constructing robust security measures. This will ultimately revolutionize patient care and outcomes.

2.6 Conclusion

Sensor-based IoT in healthcare has changed patient treatment by enabling tracking, data collection, and management from distances never conceivable previously. Among the diagnostic tools of these systems are smart diagnostic tools, ambient sensors, and wearable sensors. Their continual monitoring of health has made it possible to spot chronic conditions early. IoT has made healthcare noticeably better by improving telemedicine, smart medical equipment, and using current communication networks like 5G to communicate data more quickly. Artificial intelligence is fairly important in this context as it anticipates health trends, improves data processing, and offers customised therapeutic suggestions, improving patient outcomes. Still, the growing count of IoT devices raises serious security questions. IoT solutions have to be safe if one is to keep patient data free from illegal access and leakage. Developments in encryption systems, blockchain technology, artificial intelligence driven security solutions, and trust help reduce these risks. Designing encryption free of influence from quantum computing will be vital to protect against more threats as the technology develops. Future improvements in this field will most likely focus on allowing IoT devices to interact with one another, creating smarter AI algorithms to support more accurate diagnosis, and enhancing security procedures to protect patient data and system stability. Constantly developing sensor-based IoT, artificial intelligence, and security technologies might produce a safer, more efficient, and more tailored healthcare system. This would completely change the delivery of medical care and patient management.

References

1. Upadhyay, S.; Kumar, M.; Upadhyay, A.; Verma, S.; Kavita; Kaur, M.; Khurma, R.A.; Castillo, P.A. Challenges and Limitation Analysis of an IoT-Dependent System for Deployment in Smart Healthcare Using Communication Standards Features. *Sensors* **2023**, *23*, 5155. https://doi.org/10.3390/s23115155
2. Field, Marilyn J., ed. "Telemedicine: A guide to assessing telecommunications for health care." (1996).

3. MacKenzie, D., and J. Wajcman. "The social shaping of technology, (Open University Press, Buckingham)." (1999).
4. Ashton, Kevin. "That 'internet of things' thing." *RFID journal* 22, no. 7 (2009): 97–114.
5. Apple Inc. (2023). Apple Watch Series. Retrieved from https://www.apple.com/apple-watch-series
6. Kuzlo, Ivan, Anastasiia Strielkina, Artem Tetskyi, and Dmytro Uzun. "Selecting Cloud Service for Healthcare Applications: From Hardware to Cloud Across Machine Learning." In PhD@ ICTERI, pp. 26–34. 2018.
7. Parker, Mitchell. "Managing threats to health data and information: toward security." In Health Information Exchange, pp. 149–196. Academic, 2023.
8. Aghdam, Zahra Nasiri, Amir Masoud Rahmani, and Mehdi Hosseinzadeh. "The role of the Internet of Things in healthcare: Future trends and challenges." *Computer methods and programs in biomedicine* 199 (2021): 105903.
9. Elayan, H., Shubair, R. M., & Kiourti, A. (2017, March). Wireless sensors for medical applications: Current status and future challenges. In *2017 11th European conference on antennas and propagation (EUCAP)* (pp. 2478–2482). IEEE.
10. Vaghasiya, J.V., Mayorga-Martinez, C.C. & Pumera, M. Wearable sensors for telehealth based on emerging materials and nanoarchitectonics. *npj Flex Electron* **7**, 26 (2023). https://doi.org/10.1038/s41528-023-00261-4
11. Swan, Melanie. "Sensor mania! the internet of things, wearable computing, objective metrics, and the quantified self 2.0." *Journal of Sensor and Actuator networks* 1, no. 3 (2012): 217–253.
12. Kim, Dohyung, Jinwoo Lee, Moo Kyun Park, and Seung Hwan Ko. "Recent developments in wearable breath sensors for healthcare monitoring." *Communications Materials* 5, no. 1 (2024): 41.
13. World Health Organization (WHO). (2023). Chronic Disease Management. Retrieved from https://www.who.int/chronic_diseases
14. Qi, Jun, Po Yang, Geyong Min, Oliver Amft, Feng Dong, and Lida Xu. "Advanced internet of things for personalised healthcare systems: A survey." *Pervasive and mobile computing* 41 (2017): 132–149.
15. Topol, Eric. Deep medicine: how artificial intelligence can make healthcare human again. Hachette UK, 2019.
16. IBM Watson Health. (2020). IBM Watson Health Overview. Retrieved from https://www.ibm.com/watson-health
17. Park, Hyun-Jun, and Kyounghee Lee. "Implementation of an open artificial intelligence platform based on web and tensorflow." Journal of information and communication convergence engineering 18, no. 3 (2020): 176–182.
18. Nezhad, Mahmoud Zahedian, Ali Javan Jafari Bojnordi, Mohammad Mehraeen, Rouholla Bagheri, and Javad Rezazadeh. "Securing the future of IoT-healthcare systems: A meta-synthesis of mandatory security requirements." International Journal of Medical Informatics (2024): 105379.
19. Shah, Imdad Ali, N. Z. Jhanjhi, and Sarfraz Nawaz Brohi. "IoT Smart Healthcare Security Challenges and Solutions." In *Advances in Computational Intelligence for the Healthcare Industry 4.0*, pp. 234–247. IGI Global, 2024.
20. Haleem, Abid, Mohd Javaid, Ravi Pratap Singh, and Rajiv Suman. "Medical 4.0 technologies for healthcare: Features, capabilities, and applications." Internet of Things and Cyber-Physical Systems 2 (2022): 12–30.
21. Halamka, John, Ari Juels, Adam Stubblefield, and Jonathan Westhues. "The security implications of VeriChip cloning." *Journal of the American Medical Informatics Association* 13, no. 6 (2006): 601–607.
22. Martikainen, S. (2015). Towards better usability: Usability and end-user participation in healthcare information technology systems development (Doctoral dissertation, Itä-Suomen yliopisto).

23. Wang, Shangping, Dan Zhang, and Yaling Zhang. "Blockchain-based personal health records sharing scheme with data integrity verifiable." IEEE Access 7 (2019): 102887–102901.
24. Sarker, Sree Pradip Kumer, and Raza Zahir Khan. "Cybersecurity Considerations for Smart Bangladesh: Challenges and Solutions." Asian Journal of Research in Computer Science 17, no. 6 (2024): 145–156.
25. Syed, Naeem Firdous, Syed W. Shah, Arash Shaghaghi, Adnan Anwar, Zubair Baig, and Robin Doss. "Zero trust architecture (zta): A comprehensive survey." *IEEE Access* 10 (2022): 57143–57179.
26. Fernandez-Carames, Tiago M., and Paula Fraga-Lamas. "Towards post-quantum blockchain: A review on blockchain cryptography resistant to quantum computing attacks." *IEEE access* 8 (2020): 21091–21116.
27. Miettinen, Markus, Paul C. van Oorschot, and Ahmad-Reza Sadeghi. "Baseline functionality for security and control of commodity iot devices and domain-controlled device lifecycle management." *arXiv preprint arXiv:1808.03071* (2018).
28. Zhang, Aiqing, and Xiaodong Lin. "Towards secure and privacy-preserving data sharing in e-health systems via consortium blockchain." *Journal of medical systems* 42, no. 8 (2018): 140.
29. Bernstein, Daniel J., and Tanja Lange. "Post-quantum cryptography." *Nature* 549, no. 7671 (2017): 188–194.

Chapter 3
Cybersecurity Risks and Threats in Healthcare

Contents

Abstract Cyber security attacks on healthcare facilities are on the rise, and the increasing use of technology in day-to-day life, subsequently in the healthcare sector, has only provided more opportunities for hackers to gain and misuse patient healthcare information for personal benefits. The use of Electronic Health Records (EHR) and health information exchange opens new avenues for patient data to be accessed, used, and disclosed by cyber criminals. With the increase in cyber-attacks on the healthcare system, it's time for healthcare organizations to work towards building a strong cyber defense system. As discussed further in this paper, we will make an attempt to enlighten current cyber-attack threats on the healthcare system, the current scenario of security in the healthcare system, and some recommendations to improve the existing security system. Cyber security threats pose a major risk to efforts to integrate and improve patient care through the use of EHRs and Health Information Exchange (HIE). The potential security risks have been recognized by relevant authorities, including the US government. There have been steps to rectify the problem of security in EHRs. However, despite addressing the areas of

S. Gupta et al., *Artificial Intelligence-Enabled Security for Healthcare Systems*,
https://doi.org/10.1007/978-3-031-82810-2_3

patient privacy and electronic storage of patient data, they have not yet made sufficient effort to address the evolving nature of cyber threats and the potential hazards to patient safety and data availability. The pace of technological advancement in the healthcare system has left the security system in the dust, and healthcare systems are unable to cope with the highly sophisticated and well-resourced cyber-attack organizations. Cyber-attacks are becoming increasingly detrimental to patient healthcare, not just in privacy issues, data availability, and data integrity, but also in the potential to harm patients. For example, a patient who has had his medical records altered by a cyber-attack may receive incorrect treatment or prescriptions, having a potentially harmful effect on his health. Current common cyber security threats in healthcare include ransomware, malware, and internal data breaches by malicious intent or human error. A case in point is the 2019 attack on a clinical research organization in India. The attack was planned and executed by hacking the email account of a company executive and sending an email with a malicious attachment disguised as a quotation for construction equipment. An employee of the organization opened the said email and downloaded the compromised file, releasing NetWire malware into the company network. Subsequently, attackers were able to access the database server containing sensitive patient health information. This incident demonstrates the sophisticated nature of cyber-attacks and the potentially damaging consequences to patient healthcare.

Keywords Cyber security attacks · Healthcare facilities · Electronic health records (EHR) · Health information exchange (HIE) · Patient healthcare information · Cyber defense system

3.1 Introduction

The emergence of modern technology into various sectors has created several advancements in the working environment. In healthcare, the implementation of modern technologies such as medical devices and health information systems has offered huge benefits, for instance improved patient care and efficient management of patient data. However, the dependence on information technology (IT) has made healthcare sectors more vulnerable to various security threats. Cybersecurity and patient safety are inextricably linked. The widespread computerization of health information has resulted in substantial benefits, but there are growing concerns about the security of the information contained within electronic records. A breach of confidential patient information can have serious negative effects for patients, ranging from discrimination to damage to insurability, and in the worst cases, to identity theft. The effect of a security breach can also have a serious impact on an organization that is responsible for compromise in patient information. In addition to substantial costs, loss of patient confidence and trust may have a lasting effect on an organization's reputation.

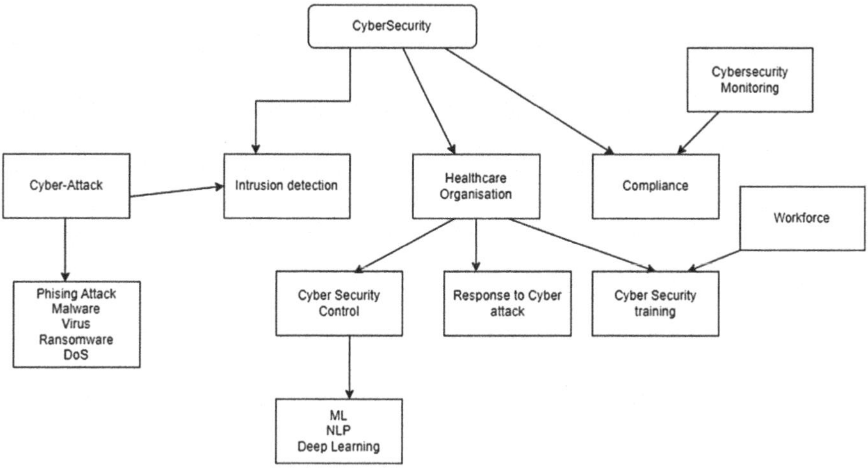

Fig. 3.1 Healthcare cybersecurity blockdiagram

Figure 3.1. has shown the growth of the internet has transformed the healthcare sector, connecting hospitals to insurance companies and patients' homes to doctors [1]. This has provided convenience and efficiency, but these developments have also created opportunities for malicious attacks on a system from internal and external sources. These attacks often are intended to access, change, or destroy electronic information [2]. Many different types of organizations are involved in healthcare, and a patient's records may end up being processed by any one of them [3]. The lack of a unified security system for healthcare data increases the risk that information in an electronic format will be vulnerable to breaches in privacy. This paper aims to explore the emerging cybersecurity risks and current vulnerabilities that are present in healthcare IT systems [4–5]. It provides an overview of the current state of security in information systems, data security, and cybersecurity practices. This paper identifies the potential impact of cyber-attacks on patient safety and offers some strategies that might help to improve the safety and security of healthcare information [6].

3.2 Extensive Literature Review Comparing and Analyzing Relevant Studies

Cybersecurity is a much greater challenge in the healthcare industry compared to any other industry, as evidenced by recent studies [7]. In a comprehensive analysis conducted across five different sectors, it was specifically discovered that healthcare had the highest cost associated with a data breach. On average, the cost amounted to a staggering \$408 per record, which is more than 2.5 times higher than the average cost faced by other industries [1, 8]. The surge in digitization within the medical field has undoubtedly brought numerous advantages, such as the convenient access and sharing of vital information [9]. However, this transition towards networked information systems has also left the healthcare sector increasingly vulnerable to security breaches. In a survey conducted on various healthcare organizations in the United States, alarming results surfaced [10–11]. Approximately 81% of these organizations admitted to experiencing at least one breach within the past 2 years. More troublingly, 16% of these organizations reported significant detrimental effects resulting from these breaches [2, 12, 13]. The frequency and severity of attacks on healthcare institutions have witnessed a significant rise between the years 2015–2016 [14]. Notably, two of the most notable breaches occurred at Anthem and Premera Blue Cross, compromising a staggering 78.8 million and 11 million patient records, respectively [3]. These incidents underscore the urgent need to comprehend the security risks that loom over the healthcare industry, in order to ensure the utmost protection of sensitive patient information [1, 15].

3.3 Overview of Cybersecurity Risks and Threats

The types of cyber-attacks and the potential risks, threats, and vulnerabilities to the health care industry are vast, as are the measures to defend against them. Cyber-attacks on the healthcare industry can be grouped into two basic categories, based on the intent of the attacker. The first category encompasses a wide range of malicious acts, the primary purpose of which is to disable a computer system or network, the most common example being denial of service (DoS) or distributed denial of service (DDoS) attacks. The second category more specifically targets unauthorized access to electronic systems or data with the intent to acquire, manipulate, or destroy sensitive information. Such attacks often seek to extort money from their victims, as in the case of the recent ransomware epidemic. It is often the case that the primary intent of the attacker influences the nature of the threat, for example one study on security breaches in the USA healthcare sector found that the highest percentage of threats (35.3%) were posed by individuals seeking to obtain personal information, this was closely followed by instances of healthcare fraud (31.8%) typically involving the intentional falsification of medical records. Due to the confidentiality and sensitivity of patient information, when it comes to cybersecurity, data security is paramount to ensure data is not leaked or disclosed to unauthorized persons. Various types of patient information with different formats and locations are held or shared throughout many healthcare systems and the complexity of these systems is often overlooked as a major threat to data security [16]. High-value information assets such as medical records and intellectual property are at risk from information theft and often there are legal obligations to protect such information from deliberate or inadvertent disclosure. Changing dynamics in the use, storage, and communication of data increase the likelihood that information may be destroyed or corrupted. We allude here to the transition from traditional paper-based

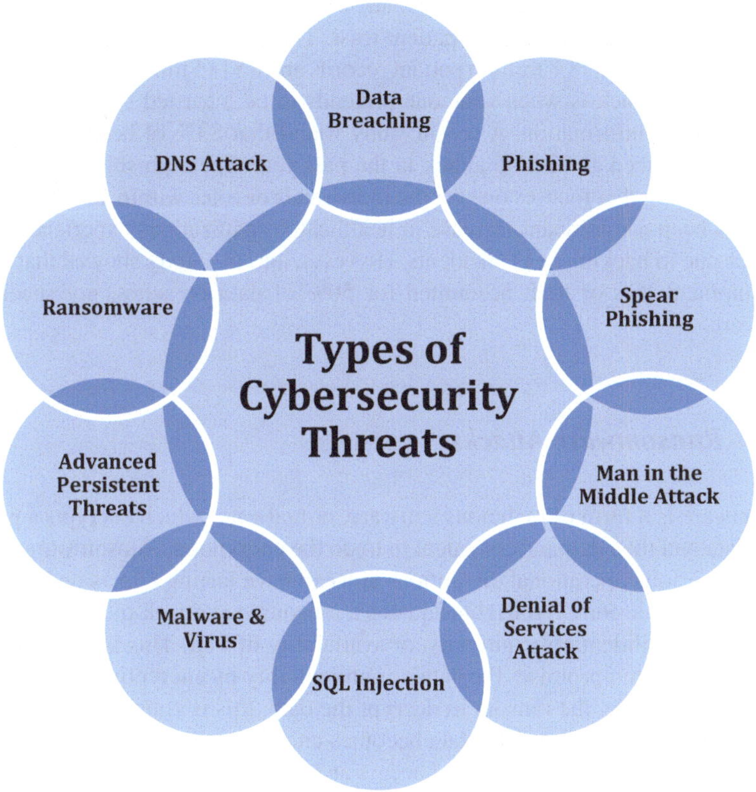

Fig. 3.2 Types of cybersecurity attack

systems to modern EHRs, which has opened up a whole new frontier for cyber-attacks, not least the aforementioned ransomware attacks. In a recent international case study for Australia and the USA, the increased use of EHRs and subsequent legal obligations were identified as a major factor contributing to the complexity of data security and the probability of data loss in these two countries. EHRs are only one example, and it is likely that future trends in healthcare IT will continue to raise the bar in terms of what is at risk and the nature of the threats posed [17]. Figure 3.2 shows various types of cybersecurity threats.

3.4 Data Breaches

Health information is often misused, leading to various breaches in security, privacy, or confidentiality. Data breaches are the most common type of system security breach, comprising 38% of all incidents reported. These breaches can have serious consequences for healthcare providers, such as legal and financial repercussions, damage to reputation, and loss of patient trust. The attack on Anthem Inc. resulted in the compromise of 78.8 million patient records and a $115 million settlement [18].

A phishing attack is when someone pretends to be a trusted source in order to obtain personal information. A recent study found that 83% of healthcare professionals experienced a phishing attack in the past year. Spear-phishing is a targeted form of phishing that focuses on specific individuals or roles within an organization. There has been a significant increase in healthcare organizations experiencing data breaches due to hacking or IT incidents. However, another study showed that physical equipment loss or theft accounted for 50% of data breaches, not specific to healthcare.

3.4.1 Ransomware Attacks

Ransomware is a form of malicious software, or malware, which encrypts a participant's data and then demands payment to undo the encryption. Ransomware attacks can cause serious operational disruptions and can have lasting effects on an organization. The Office for Civil Rights equates a ransomware attack to a data breach if it affects the confidentiality, integrity, or availability of PHI. This is because a ransomware attack compromises the data's confidentiality by encrypting it. If a participant is forced to pay the ransom to decrypt the data, this is considered a breach of data integrity. And finally, if the data becomes encrypted and inaccessible to a participant, this is considered a denial of access and is also a breach of data availability. Ransomware has become an increasingly pervasive form of cyber attack, leading to a more concerted effort to prevent and combat these attacks, and creating a greater amount of resources available to those affected [19].

An example of a ransomware attack in healthcare is an event that affected the Hollywood Presbyterian Medical Center, where the entire medical center essentially ground to a halt after an infection of malware caused the data on its computer systems to become encrypted and inaccessible. The attackers demanded an exorbitant amount of money to provide the medical center with the decryption key to unlock the data.

In response to the increasing prevalence and detrimental effects of ransomware attacks, the HHS has released a new set of HIPAA guidelines. In the event of a ransomware attack, the HHS recommends the affected organization to treat it as an incident involving PHI data loss, and to act in accordance with HIPAA breach notification procedures. The HHS also advises organizations to conduct regular data backups to ensure the integrity and availability of their data, as well as have a well-thought-out contingency plan for the restoration of lost data.

3.4.2 Phishing and Social Engineering

Phishing and social engineering strategies are particularly important to detect and avoid since they rely on human error and prediction, rather than technical vulnerabilities in the systems. Phishing is a targeted attack on an individual to trick them into revealing sensitive information or to install malware on their computer. It often aims to steal login details or to capture information such as credit card numbers. The attack in healthcare is very prevalent due to the number of access points to valuable personal data, computer systems are often used by many individuals, hard to track and the nature of clinical work requires quick and easy access to data. Typical examples are impersonation of staff to gain information about patients, sending emails posing as an authoritative figure to get an employee to reveal information or to change their payroll information, and posing as an IT vendor with the intent of installing malware. With large numbers of staff working irregular hours in a high-stress environment, it can be difficult to remind everyone of these types of attack and to remain vigilant against them. An Alberta Health Services employee received a phishing email and entered their network credentials, after which the email account started sending out more phishing emails to other staff. A malware strain known as Dyre was involved in a cyber-attack that netted cybercriminals over 121,000 USD from a Kentucky hospital, the malware began when an employee opened a phishing email and proceeded to capture logins for online bank accounts. Dyre was also behind a recent attack on the Southlake Regional Health Centre in Newmarket, Ontario where an employee clicked a link in an email and installed the malware, this caused the IT department to take their system offline in fear that patient data was being compromised. Dyre has the potential to cause vast financial loss due to online banking fraud [20].

3.4.3 Malware and Viruses

Early forms of malware, such as viruses and worms, entered into the realm of healthcare for one of the same purposes it did in other industries: the ability to wreak havoc and cause despair. Once again, with the sole purpose of destruction or as part of a paid deal (to disrupt services so that certain companies can fix the problem). A very well-known example that affected many NHS hospitals in the United Kingdom during 2017 was the WannaCry ransomware cryptoworm. After becoming infected, the worm encrypts data and demands payment using bitcoin. The worm itself was created and distributed using an exploit on Microsoft Windows operating system. Throughout 2017 and 2018, the worm had resurfaced and caused havoc within the healthcare sector. Another form of malware is spyware, which is designed to stealthily obtain data from a computing device without the user's knowledge. Spyware can arrive at the hands of healthcare providers unwittingly installed on a work computer, and it can severely breach doctor-patient confidentiality.

Finally, adware, often seen in the forms of pop-ups, can be used to gather information on a patient for a variety of reasons. All of these malware types can be implemented very easily and are highly effective within a sector that predominantly uses computer systems.

As a direct consequence of the complexities in healthcare technology, including EPR, many various medical devices, global healthcare services, and many more, malware has proven itself as a high-severity threat. As touched on earlier, this is largely due to the wide variety of patients and services malware seeks to damage or exploit. Specifically, in EPR and the storage of patient data, malware has the potential to do irreversible damage to databases and corrupt or delete patient information. In the case where EPR has a version of patient treatment plans, a critical patient's continuity of care may be disrupted. Results of diagnostic tests and medical images stored digitally are also at high risk of data loss, which can affect patient care. Throughout the last two decades, it has been highly documented the risk of internet-connected medical devices being targeted for cyber-attacks. This threat only increases as technology advances. An accurate example from 2017 stated that a global cyber-attack using NSA exploits had caused a shutdown of GE medical devices in a specific area of US healthcare. This method of malware exploitation on medical devices can greatly affect services and the safety of patients.

3.4.4 Insider Threats

The threat from insiders is considered one of the most dangerous. The Cyber Security Intelligence Index, 2015, states that 55% of all attacks were carried out by insiders. The categorization of an 'insider' can be from a member of staff, a contractor or business associate who has access to the organization's system. Insiders have knowledge of the systems and potentially how to cause maximum damage. Disgruntled employees may perform acts which they have been planning for a long time, using their knowledge of the system to access information which they are unauthorized to access, with the intention of damaging their organization. Due to the nature of healthcare and the sensitive information it handles, it is more likely to be the victim of targeted attacks from malicious insiders. Data protection is a key priority for the NHS. It is reportedly spending £20 million in 2016 to improve data security, in response to recent high-profile attacks. A recent example was the case of a locum doctor who was able to access over 1000 patient records in an eight-day period. He was able to access information unrelated to the care he was providing and his activities were identified as suspicious by the surgery staff. The surgery had not restricted his access to the system sufficiently. He was fined £300 and the case was taken to court, where he was ordered to pay the prosecution £990, a victim surcharge of £60 and the cost of £864.63. This shows that the Information Commissioner's Office is willing to take legal action against those who breach patient confidentiality. In the doctor's case, he faced emotional stress and the loss of his job. Although this may generally be a light punishment, the fines given for data breaches from EU's General Data Protection Regulation will be much larger, this is set to be enforced from mid-2018 depending on the UK's position following Brexit [21].

3.5 Case Studies of High-Profile Cybersecurity Incidents

The healthcare industry in the United States has been slow to respond to the growing threat of cyber-attacks (Coiera, 2016). Although the types of attack, extent of damage, and overall impact in healthcare can be difficult to fully measure due to variations of reporting, there have been a few high-profile cases which have been well documented in recent years. These case studies offer an important insight into the types of cyber-attacks targeting the healthcare industry and their potential impacts [22].

WannaCry ransomware attack, in May 2017, the WannaCry ransomware crypto-worm was unleashed upon the world. The worm targeted computers running the Microsoft Windows operating system by encrypting data and demanding ransom payment in Bitcoin cryptocurrency. WannaCry was particularly ill-timed for the UK's National Health Service and other international health organisations. The worm took advantage of a Windows SMB protocol vulnerability to spread itself within affected networks. This incident exacerbated existing infrastructure problems within the NHS and ultimately led to the cancellation of an estimated 19,500 medical appointments—including 139 potential cancer referrals. A kill switch to stop the spread of the worm was found by an accidental hero but not before WannaCry had made global impact infecting an estimated 200,000 computers across 150 countries and causing hundreds of millions of dollars in damages. The US and UK attributed the attack to North Korean hacking group Lazarus. This was a clear example of how a common type of malware can have widespread impact when systems are not kept up-to-date with security patches [23].

The Department of Veterans Affairs in the US experienced one of the worst known breaches of personal data when in 2006 a laptop was stolen from an employee's home which contained the personal information of 26.5 million veterans and military personnel. The information included names, social security numbers, and dates of birth. The laptop was later recovered and determined to have been stolen as part of a routine burglary with the perpetrator having no knowledge of the value of the data. It was confirmed that the sensitive data had not been the target of the theft or accessed in any way, so it was hailed as one of the rarest cases in security breaches where information was not misused. However, the VA's handling of the incident was heavily criticised. An information security program was already underway at the VA, but an investigation found that the data had not been included in the program's security certification and accreditation process. This led to widespread criticism of the VA's information security and ultimately a security overhaul and new legislation enhancing data security for veterans. [24]

3.5.1 *WannaCry Ransomware Attack*

Back in May 12th, 2017, WannaCry ransomware, which is also called WannaCrypt, WanaCrypt0r 2.0, Wanna Decryptor, infected 230,000 computers all over 150 countries. The ransomware encrypts the files and demands ransom payments in the form of $300 in Bitcoins. The attack leaked over 20 percent or 10,000 of NHS (National Health Service) England's computers have been infected by the ransomware, which disrupted appointments and forced the NHS to turn away patients until the issues were resolved. The outcome from this attack puts the patients' lives in critical condition at the moment. Since the severity impact of the attack, NHS England declared the ransomware attack as a major incident. A major incident is an event that leads to a significant impact on the NHS, requiring an increase in the level of response and specific arrangements. Although a crisis happened in the NHS due to the ransomware attack, the Health Secretary at the time, Jeremy Hunt, confirmed that there has not been any evidence or reports regarding patient data being breached from the cyber attack. This ransomware attack has proven that NHS digital assets are highly critical and valuable in the cyber world. However, the ransomware attack affects medical devices such as MRI scanners that run outdated operating systems such as Windows XP, which could make the devices vulnerable to these types of attacks. [25]

3.5.2 *NotPetya Malware Attack*

The NotPetya malware attack occurred in July 2017 and had a significant impact on the healthcare sector. NotPetya, a variant of the Petya ransomware, initially spread through a compromised update to M.E.Doc accounting software. It had rapid lateral movement thanks to the use of EternalBlue and EternalRomance SMB exploits. Although it encrypted files as typical ransomware, the failure to provide a means of decryption meant that paying a ransom would not result in file recovery. Restoration of files from backup was also not a feasible option, as NotPetya's use of a modified boot sector meant that even if files were decrypted, they would be in an unusable state. This had severe consequences for healthcare organizations who were not only unable to access patient data required for treatment but also faced a legal requirement to report data breaches involving loss of access to this data. In the case of NHS England, 19,500 medical appointments were canceled, and the cost of the attack was later estimated to be £92 million. However, this did not account for the longer-term effects on the organization. The head of the UK's National Cyber Security Centre described the event as "indiscriminate exploitation for a criminal act". It had been launched with no intent to affect the NHS [23].

3.5.3 Anthem Data Breach

On February 4, 2015, health insurer Anthem, Inc. reported that their database had been hacked, which resulted in an infiltration compromising 78.8 million people's records. The attackers gained access to names, birthdays, medical IDs, social security numbers, street addresses, email addresses, and employment information including income and employer. It is considered to be the largest data breach in the healthcare sector to date. According to Joseph Swedish, the company's CEO, "These attackers gained unauthorized access to Anthem's IT system and have obtained personal information from our current and former members such as their names, birthdays, medical IDs/social security numbers, street addresses, email addresses, and employment information including income." This incident prompted Swedish to issue an apology to customers and to vigorously look into the situation in order to remediate it. Although there is currently no evidence that the data has been used maliciously, it is likely to end up on the black market and buy and sell medical information. Due to the sensitivity of this type of data, affected customers are now subject to a high risk of identity theft and fraud. A lawsuit has been filed in California accusing Anthem of failing to protect sensitive information. Anthem is offering 2 years of identity theft repair assistance to affected customers. This is a prime example of the risk that the digital age poses on our personal information [26].

3.5.4 Community Health Systems Data Breach

As an organization, Community Health Systems reported the theft of patient data in 2014. According to reports, attackers belonging to the Advanced Persistent Threat group stole approximately 4.5 million patients' names, Social Security numbers, addresses, birthdays, and telephone numbers by bypassing the company's security measures. The attack was discovered first in April, but it is assumed the breach began in July or August 2013. FireEye's report on the matter states that the attackers used malware and technology that was undetectable by IT personnel and took an approximate 6-week period to install and retrieve information before any action was taken to remove it. At least 2 servers were used that were previously dormant, and it is unsure whether they were a part of the CHS system or of another data storage site. The methods used in this attack were incredibly well planned and executed, taking into account that the attackers were not interested in any other form of information other than patient data. This instance alone resulted in a significant monetary loss for CHS. However, in the larger scheme of healthcare, it sets a substantial example of how the value of patient information has now made the healthcare industry a very lucrative target for cyber attacks [27].

3.5.5 Equifax Data Breach

The Equifax data breach occurred between May and July 2017. The breach was not made public until September, when Equifax stated that it had discovered the breach on July 29. It is estimated that 143 million Americans' social security numbers were exposed and that 44 million British residents may have also been affected. The breach is thought to have occurred due to a vulnerability in Apache Struts, the fix for which was issued on March 6. This has led to criticism of Equifax's handling of public disclosure regarding the breach, as a patch could have been implemented immediately after its release to prevent the breach occurring. Equifax's stock price fell by more than 30% after the announcement of the breach. The company has subsequently been involved in several lawsuits on behalf of those affected by the breach. As of September 26, the US Congress has moved to repeal a rule that would have allowed consumers to file class action lawsuits against financial companies. In the wake of the breach, Equifax put out a statement that its CEO, Richard Smith, would retire. This breach is indicative of the increasing threat to private data by cyber criminal activity. With the large quantity of sensitive information now being stored digitally, the potential benefits to cyber criminals of attacking such a database greatly outweigh the costs of investing in more sophisticated forms of malware. In this case, the sensitive nature and high volume of data held by Equifax made it a significant target [28].

3.6 Impact of Cyber-Attacks on Patient Outcomes

In section "7. Impact of cyber-attacks on patient outcomes," it is discussed that the study by Fritz and colleagues found that hospitals who experienced a breach had a longer average length of stay and were specifically associated with adverse events. This can have substantial financial implications by way of Medicare reimbursement penalties for hospital-acquired conditions and can increase malpractice liability if patients experience harm. One study in a UK NHS hospital found that a malware cyber-attack can disrupt the blood transfusion process and lead to "10,000 errors in tracking the patients' blood transfusion status, including delays to care and blood transfusion near-misses." This shows how patient safety can be severely compromised and result in harmful medical errors with potential long-term consequences. In a study conducted by Sittig and Singh, they described how certain types of health IT are involved in more than a thousand patient deaths [29]. Various Cybersecurity impacts on patient is shown in Fig. 3.3.

This gap in adverse event and mortality research related to cyber-attacks using detailed case studies has been identified as a critical area where future researchers can help quantify the potential harms to patients. A recent study has found that data

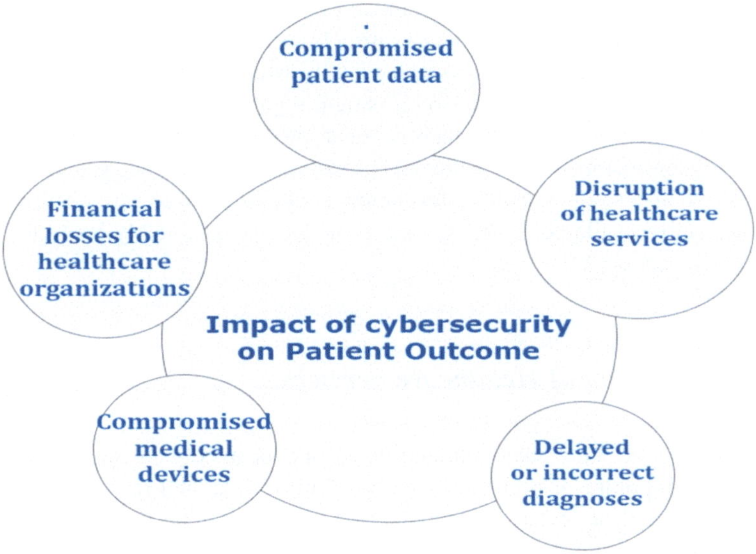

Fig. 3.3 Impact of cybersecurity on patient outcome

breaches were associated with a significant increase in mortality in the years following the breach, with breaches in facilities with a poor grade on patient safety being at the highest risk. By understanding the magnitude of adverse event and mortality increases over the long term and the specific mechanisms by which these events occur, it will be possible to formulate and test targeted interventions to mitigate these harms and prevent future incidents from occurring [30].

3.6.1 Compromised Patient Data

The healthcare industry relies on patient information to provide care effectively. Protection of patient data is an essential mission involving a sense of individual privacy and a well-functioning healthcare system. Nonetheless, with advances in technology, the confidentiality and security of patient information has become more elusive. The potential impact on patient data disclosure by the healthcare provider can have a detrimental effect on patient safety and quality of care. Patient data are a lucrative target for attackers, making healthcare providers prime targets for data theft. Personal health information contains a wealth of data elements making identity theft a useful crime. Other motives for attacking patient data include competitive intelligence, insurance fraud, and in rare cases, infliction of harm on an individual [31]. Consider the wealth of available patient data and the multiple access points between providers, insurance companies, and supporting administrative systems. It is hard to detect a patient data security breach, and it may happen more than once. Health systems are not always immediately aware of breaches of patient data; they may be contacted much later by a patient regarding a case of identity theft. Data leakage can occur if health data is not encrypted when sent to an offsite backup service. Subcontractors of any health data processing can introduce yet another vector of data theft. Personal health information can be difficult to safeguard in that it must be readily available to the service provider yet adequately protected from unwarranted access [32].

3.6.2 Disruption of Healthcare Services

Cyber-attacks can cause major disruption to healthcare organizations. This may involve the temporary or permanent loss of clinical data, and in severe cases, the corruption of medical devices. Disruption of healthcare can have a major impact on patient safety and care. Attacks may limit access to essential data or cause damage to medical devices, putting patients at risk. In 2017, the WannaCry ransomware attack had a major impact on the NHS, with an estimated 19,000 appointments cancelled as a result of the attack. The virus took advantage of vulnerabilities in Windows operating systems, encrypting data and demanding ransoms for its return. The attack led to a third of NHS trusts being disrupted and had long-lasting impacts on some services. This is a good example of how vulnerabilities in IT systems can be exploited to cause immediate disruption to healthcare [33].

3.6.3 Delayed or Incorrect Diagnoses

When healthcare information is unavailable due to system downtime or data loss, patients may find themselves receiving a delayed diagnosis or one that is "off the mark." This is dangerous, particularly in cases where a condition is life-threatening, such as cancer or a heart condition [34]. If the healthcare provider or patient is unable to access previous medical history, allergy information, or prescription drug information, then the chances of making an incorrect diagnosis increases. Unavailability of data can also lead to more tests being ordered, which can be costly and time-consuming for the patient. If the tests cannot be analyzed or the results are lost, this may require the patient to undergo the same tests again. All of these problems can stem from system downtime, incompatibility of systems, or inadequate information availability, all of which are issues that arise from poor cybersecurity in healthcare [35].

3.6.4 Compromised Medical Devices

Many healthcare operations have become automated, and this increases the potential risk for cyber-attacks. Medical devices are now built with internet access in mind for ease of updates, data transmission, and interconnectivity within the healthcare industry. The range of medical devices includes implantable devices (such as cardiac pacemakers) to large-scale imaging systems (such as MRI scanners). Both of these devices have more complex data usage and transfer, and if compromised, have greater implications for patient safety.

With the increased requirements for real-time information and availability for the purposes of safety and patient outcomes, cloud computing is an attractive option within the healthcare industry. The scale of data among healthcare enterprises is very large, and the cost for storage is often too expensive. Cloud computing offers a potential cost reduction of data storage. This has the potential to benefit healthcare with medical research and accessibility of patient data for the administration of care. However, the implications of cloud computing have a large impact on data security. With data becoming virtualized, the activity for data transfer increases, and the physical storage of data becomes unknown. Encryption methods for data protection during transfer to the cloud and while being stored are often difficult, as decryption is required for data usage in medical applications. Failure to encrypt data or improper encryption methods have the potential for data interception during data transfer to the cloud and unauthorized access to patient records. Cloud storage involves pooled data from multiple sources, the sharing of data storage, and the networking of large virtualized resources, making cloud storage an ideal target and a location with potential for large data source breaches [36].

The basic structure of computer networking within healthcare enterprises starts with internet/intranet networking infrastructure and moves down to networked medical devices and networked medical applications. As with any type of computer networking, internet and intranet networking require strong firewalling and network security measures to prevent unauthorized access from external sources. The networking of medical applications involves data transfer between medical application servers and clinician/patient computers. Any data transfer involving patient information must be secure and traceable, and failure to do so may result in a breach of patient confidentiality. However, most at risk are networked medical devices. Networked medical devices share a common use of general-purpose operating systems and standard networking protocols. Often device manufacturers aim to develop devices that can be integrated into existing network infrastructure, and devices may be left with default settings that make them insecure. An investigation by the ACMD concluded that networked medical devices often have little or no security measures in place to prevent unauthorized access. A study by KrypteX found that a selection of infusion pumps were shipped with identical embedded usernames and passwords. This means that networked medical devices are at significant risk from malware or targeted attacks, and if compromised, have the potential to serve as an access point to other areas of the network. A well-known example was the computer viruses

SQLSlammer and Blaster. These worms infected IT networks whereby unpatched devices resulted in the global propagation of these viruses within 24 hours.

3.6.5 Financial Losses for Healthcare Organizations

Financial costs related to cybersecurity risks are obviously not the most important aspect to life or limb that could hinge on the next catastrophic failure, but it is still extremely important as an issue. Costs can have direct involvement speculating from fines, loss of revenue or intellectual property all the way to the other end of the scale reducing consumer confidence in a product or healthcare provider. A healthcare organization must evaluate the likelihood of a data loss incident and the impact this will have on the organization. Data loss costs the most out of the aforementioned issues with higher education institutions reporting loss at £125 per record. This section will cover financial issues that might occur and a model will be proposed to help measure the expenditure of implementing cybersecurity measures.

The largest personalized computing device is the medical industry and is almost completely reliant on data. A common misconception is that data being unattainable is the only outcome of a cybersecurity issue when trying to attack a system and this misconception is that data is still available but just corrupted and the system issues no warning. Most methods of attacks will result in data being destroyed and being an incident that the attack has been successful and now reaching the open data theft. Data destruction can be catastrophic dependent on the type and the loss involved can also often be irreversible. An example of a type of data that if lost would be irrecoverable and result in patient care issues is the loss of electronic health records (EHR). Various information newly added to EHR systems can be critical in life-saving situations. An NHS case of a doctor's ability to cure a patient of a case of pneumonia that took a downhill turn and required hospital care was dependent on knowing which lung the infection was in. Without the patient knowing, the doctor managed to find this information and had it result in quick recovery care. Without this piece of information, the treatment could be life-threatening and there is no way to recover this specific piece of information. EHR is often used as a case to the attempt of starting to implement cost-effective security measures with the belief that the cost of loss is outweighed by costs of prevention. In the case that information is still available, data theft will result in loss of consumer confidence in where and who they are willing to receive healthcare from.

3.7 Impact of Cyber-Attacks on Healthcare Organizations

Healthcare organizations are considered a soft target for cyber-attacks due to their lack of security and their significant value of personal data. Large-scale shifts from paper to electronic health records make the healthcare sector an ideal target for hackers. In addition, medical identity theft is often not identified by the patient or provider, causing the information to be used for years without detection. Figure 3.4 shows the impact of cyber-attacks on healthcare organizations.

The type of data held by healthcare organizations also makes them a prime target. Personal health information contains a wealth of personal information that can be used for identity theft, a common MO for many cyber-attacks. The value of the data can also cause it to be held to ransom by various encryption tactics, an example being the recent spate of ransomware attacks on hospitals. Once stolen, data can be used for insurance fraud, pharmaceutical drug fraud, and the creation of fake IDs to buy medical equipment and supplies. In another angle, the alteration of medical data can have life-threatening consequences to the patient. This range of factors makes the security of patient data of paramount importance to healthcare organizations worldwide [37].

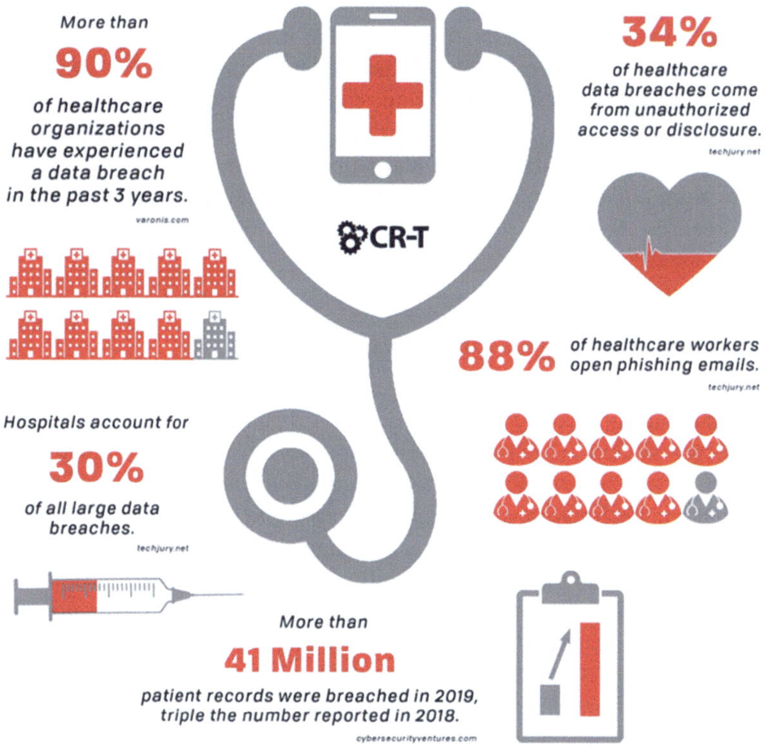

Fig. 3.4 Impact of cybersecurity on healthcare organization

3.7.1 Reputational Damage

A good hospital's reputation is built on trust that they can look after sensitive data properly and will take a dim view of any unwarranted exposure of information. Patients are fiercely protective of their medical details, and given the damage that can be done with medical identity theft, for the hospital, this is a make or break issue. When people's lives are at stake, there is a requirement for discretion, and a failure to maintain privacy can easily be perceived as a failure in the duty of care. High-profile incidents of data loss can decimate a healthcare organization's reputation, and recovery can be very difficult. If a patient feels that they can no longer trust their hospital to look after their best interests, they will take their custom elsewhere. Data breaches can also cause major legal problems, and costs arising from them add to the total damage experienced as a result of the incident [38].

Given the importance of patient data to patient welfare and the function of care providers, reputational damage is a highly significant yet often overlooked aspect of data breaches and other security incidents. Unlike a direct financial loss, there are no calculable metrics for reputation or trust, but it is widely understood that they have an enormous influence on the success of the organization. Because of this, it can be challenging to recover losses from reputational damage, and they may have a long-lasting effect. Although it is difficult to assess the precise amount of damage sustained and the value of data loss or leaks, understanding the nature of the damage will help in identifying means for preventing it and aid in the planning of cost-effective security measures.

3.7.2 Legal and Regulatory Consequences

Security in the healthcare industry is important for patient safety and the success of the healthcare system. The loss or theft of patient information or costly medical equipment can have a devastating effect on patient care and may even cause a medical error. Due to the importance of healthcare, new and complex regulatory requirements have been put in place. Because of the sensitive nature of patient information in healthcare, the Health Insurance Portability and Accountability Act (HIPAA) was implemented to ensure data privacy and security are maintained. Any organization found to be in violation of HIPAA can face civil and criminal penalties. Civil penalties can range from $100 to $50,000 per violation (or per record), with a maximum penalty of $1.5 million per year for each violation. Criminal penalties for HIPAA violations can range from $50,000 to $250,000 in fines and/or 1 to 10 years in prison. Other countries also have strict laws regarding the privacy of medical records. For example, a UK organization found to be in serious violation of the Data Protection Act can face a fine of up to £500,000. Healthcare organizations also have to consider the impact of malpractice, where an error in patient care caused by lost or unavailable patient information could result in a lawsuit. In this case, the admissibility of the breached information into evidence could have a damaging effect on the case. In the worst-case scenario where a breach has directly caused patient harm, the organization could be faced with a potential lawsuit [39].

3.7.3 Financial Impact

The financial costs of cyber-attacks in healthcare vary widely. One US study found that the average cost of a data breach was $158 per lost or stolen record, with detection, notification, and post-breach response costs also factored in. Another study reported an average consolidated cost of $3.62 million for a data breach. Malicious or criminal attacks accounted for 51% of breaches and were the most expensive. Comparing these studies, it is clear that healthcare data breaches are costly. Another study found that the healthcare industry is more susceptible to cyber-attacks compared to other industries, with data breaches in healthcare costing as much as $408 per record and as much as $2 million more than breaches in other industries [18].

3.7.4 Increased Cybersecurity Expenditures

With the evolution of cybersecurity threats and the implementation of advanced technological systems in healthcare, the cost of developing and maintaining the right cybersecurity infrastructure to protect patient data has continued to grow. Over the past few years, healthcare organizations' spending on IT has increased significantly in order to address federal requirements to implement electronic medical records (EMRs) while at the same time information security threats have also increased. This can be represented in the increase of security-related incidents in the past 2 years. According to a Deloitte 2012 report, patient data security breaches in the US cost hospitals $6 billion.

Organizations are now beginning to understand various direct and indirect costs associated with data breaches and the overall loss of data. An indirect cost could be the loss of reputation and patients to other healthcare organizations. In an age of global shared electronic health records, a patient can choose another provider down the road or in another country. According to CIO magazine, the top healthcare provider in the U.S. can lose $100 million to $300 million because of a data breach.

Direct costs could be fines and/or legal fees that are associated with an information security-related incident. One of the more highly publicized incidents in recent times is the incident regarding the British Broadcasting Corporation (BBC) and New York Presbyterian Hospital. They were fined a total of $4.8 million due to the disclosure of patient data. Measures to curb cybersecurity incidents and data loss have been reflected in the increased spending on technologies to prevent, detect, and respond. This includes encryption products, DLP solutions, stronger authentication processes, and development of more advanced and intelligent security systems. This can be summarized in a HealthcareInfoSecurity survey where 40% of respondents stated they would be increasing their budget for information security technology [40].

3.7.5 Loss of Patient Trust

Loss of patient trust often happens when sensitive information is leaked due to cyberattacks. It is very difficult to restore trust after an incident and may result in patients seeking care at other facilities, ultimately leading to loss of revenue for the affected organization. In the worst case scenario, patients may file lawsuits seeking damages for the leakage of their sensitive information. For instance, in 2014, the US hospital operator Community Health Systems had a data breach involving the personal information of about 4.5 million patients. Although there were no allegations of wrongdoing or that personal information was used inappropriately, they still face more than a dozen lawsuits with one seeking more than $4 billion in damages. This was because the trust was already lost between patients and the organization, hence they felt that their information was not safe in the hands of the organization [41].

3.8 Strategies for Mitigating Cybersecurity Risks

An effective defense strategy against cyber-attacks and risk is crucial. Human firewall training is invaluable in providing a first line of defense. Increasing awareness and having an educated workforce helps identify and respond to threats. Cost can be reduced through tools like full disk encryption. Data breaches can cost organizations millions. Encryption is important for protecting health data. Every organization with an online presence should have an incident response strategy. Organizations without a plan spend more on data breaches. The response plan includes containing the breach, assessing damage, and recovering. It should be well documented and continuously updated for better success and efficiency. [18]

3.9 Competitive Data on Cybersecurity Risks and Threats in Healthcare

In order to fully comprehend and gain a comprehensive understanding of the prevailing and ever-evolving landscape of cybersecurity risks and potential threats that plague the healthcare industry, it becomes absolutely crucial and essentially imperative to meticulously delve deep into the realm of competitive data. This intricate process helps shed light on the numerous vulnerabilities and susceptibilities that healthcare organizations across the globe often encounter, as well as the profound and far-reaching impacts that stem from these menacing challenges. It is within this understanding that we can truly grasp the exigency to prioritize and safeguard the integrity, confidentiality, and accessibility of sensitive healthcare-related information. Expanding upon this crucial need to prioritize and safeguard healthcare information, it is essential to recognize the intricate and complex nature of cybersecurity threats in the healthcare industry. With the exponential growth of technology and digital advancements, the risks and potential threats faced by healthcare organizations have become more sophisticated and widespread. Thus, it is imperative to delve deeply into the realm of competitive data in order to gain a comprehensive understanding of these risks and vulnerabilities. By meticulously analyzing this data, healthcare organizations can identify the weaknesses and susceptibilities that they may encounter, enabling them to develop robust and effective cybersecurity strategies. Moreover, by recognizing the far-reaching impacts that these challenges can have, healthcare organizations can comprehend the urgent need to prioritize the integrity, confidentiality, and accessibility of sensitive healthcare-related information. By doing so, they can ensure the safety and security of patient data, protecting it from unauthorized access, data breaches, and other potential threats. As the healthcare industry continues to evolve, so do the cybersecurity risks it faces. Therefore, staying ahead of these risks requires a continuous commitment to monitoring and analyzing competitive data, in order to remain vigilant and proactive in identifying and mitigating potential threats. Furthermore, healthcare organizations must collaborate and share knowledge across the industry, fostering a culture of information exchange and collective defense against cyber threats [2]. Only through such comprehensive understanding and collaboration can the healthcare industry effectively safeguard the privacy and security of patient information, preserving the trust and confidence of patients worldwide. By staying informed about the current trends and emerging threats in cybersecurity, healthcare organizations can effectively address the challenges they face. This involves not only understanding the technical aspects of cybersecurity, but also recognizing the human factors that contribute to vulnerabilities [7]. For example, social engineering tactics such as phishing attacks and employee negligence can expose healthcare organizations to significant risks. By educating staff members about these risks and implementing robust training programs, healthcare organizations can enhance their overall security posture [8]. Furthermore, it is essential for healthcare organizations to regularly assess their cybersecurity readiness and conduct thorough risk assessments. This includes evaluating the effectiveness of existing security controls, identifying any potential gaps or weaknesses, and implementing appropriate remediation measures. By regularly reviewing and updating their cybersecurity practices, healthcare organizations can ensure that they remain resilient in the face of evolving threats [12]. Additionally, healthcare organizations should consider adopting a proactive approach to cybersecurity by engaging in threat intelligence sharing communities and participating in cybersecurity exercises and simulations. These initiatives can help organizations improve their incident response capabilities and strengthen their defenses against potential threats. By collaborating with other industry stakeholders, healthcare organizations can gain valuable insights and leverage collective knowledge to better protect their systems and data. In conclusion, the ever-evolving landscape of cybersecurity risks and threats in the healthcare industry necessitates a comprehensive and proactive approach to safeguarding sensitive information. By delving deep into the realm of competitive data, healthcare organizations can gain a thorough understanding of the vulnerabilities they face and develop effective strategies to mitigate risks. Through collaboration, knowledge sharing, and continuous monitoring, the healthcare industry can fortify its defenses against cybersecurity threats and ensure the privacy and security of patient information [22]. Table 3.1 shows a brief overview on competitive data on cybersecurity risks and threats in healthcare.

Table 3.1 Competitive data on cybersecurity risks and threats in healthcare

Category	Threat actors	Examples	Impact	Mitigation strategies
Data Breaches	Hackers, cybercriminals, insiders	Large-scale ransomware attacks targeting healthcare providers. Phishing campaigns targeting healthcare staff. Insider threats involving unauthorized access by employees.	Loss of patient trust and reputation damage. Financial penalties for HIPAA violations. Disruption of healthcare operations.	Implement strong access controls and data encryption. Regularly train staff on cybersecurity awareness. Deploy intrusion detection and prevention systems.
Denial-of-Service (DoS) Attacks	Hacktivists, cybercriminals	DoS attacks targeting hospital networks, disrupting patient care. DoS attacks targeting appointment booking systems.	Disruption of critical healthcare services. Delayed or cancelled medical procedures. Loss of revenue for healthcare providers.	Implement DDoS mitigation strategies. Increase network redundancy and capacity. Develop incident response plans for DoS attacks.
Malware and Ransomware	Cybercriminals, organized crime groups	Ransomware attacks on hospitals, forcing them to pay to regain access to critical data. Malware targeting medical devices, disrupting their functionality.	Disruption of healthcare operations and patient care. Financial losses due to ransom payments. Potential harm to patients if medical devices are compromised.	Implement endpoint protection software and firewalls. Regularly update software and firmware on devices. Back up data regularly and ensure backups are secure.

(continued)

Table 3.1 (continued)

Category	Threat actors	Examples	Impact	Mitigation strategies
Supply Chain Attacks	Nation-state actors, cybercriminals	Compromised software updates from a medical device vendor. Hacking into a cloud service provider used by a healthcare organization.	Indirect access to healthcare systems and patient data. Potential disruption of healthcare operations. Reputational damage for healthcare providers.	Conduct thorough security assessments of third-party vendors. Negotiate strong security clauses in contracts with vendors. Monitor third-party activity for suspicious behavior.
Social Engineering Attacks	Phishing scammers, social engineers	Phishing emails targeting healthcare staff to gain access to login credentials. Social engineering attacks impersonating IT personnel to gain access to systems.	Data breaches and unauthorized access to healthcare systems. Financial losses due to fraudulent activities. Erosion of patient trust.	Regularly train staff on social engineering tactics. Implement multi-factor authentication for accessing sensitive systems. Foster a culture of cybersecurity awareness among staff.

3.10 Conclusion

The healthcare sector has entered a new era of digital medicine. This era promises to bring many benefits to patients, practitioners, and those involved in the healthcare process. Information and technologies in digital medicine are tools to be used in a complex adaptive system. It should be realized that introducing IT to healthcare may cause both expected and unanticipated changes to complex adaptive systems. Much work needs to be done to understand what these changes are and how IT implementation can be used to steer these changes in a positive direction. This report has identified risks and threats to the security of healthcare data and information due to IT implementation in the healthcare sector [12]. The risks identified include endangerment of patient safety, privacy, quality of care, increased cost of liability, compromised data integrity, impact on the availability of healthcare services, and the costs of IT implementation and maintenance. Numerous vulnerabilities in today's healthcare IT infrastructure, which might lead to security breaches, have also been outlined in this report. These two factors combined present a formidable challenge to maintaining the security of healthcare data and information in the digital age and raise serious concerns as to whether the benefits of IT in healthcare will outweigh the risks [37].

References

1. J. J. Hathaliya and S. Tanwar, "An exhaustive survey on security and privacy issues in Healthcare 4.0," Computer Communications, 2020. [HTML]
2. A. Attaallah, H. Alsuhabi, S. Shukla, "Analyzing the Big Data Security Through a Unified Decision-Making Approach," in Computer Automation & Soft Computing, 2022. semanticscholar.org
3. S. R. Oh, Y. D. Seo, E. Lee, and Y. G. Kim, "A comprehensive survey on security and privacy for electronic health data," International Journal of Environmental Research and Public Health, 2021, mdpi.com. mdpi.com
4. C. Butpheng, K. H. Yeh, and H. Xiong, "Security and privacy in IoT-cloud-based e-health systems—A comprehensive review," Symmetry, 2020. mdpi.com
5. A. López Martínez, M. Gil Pérez, et al., "A comprehensive review of the state-of-the-art on security and privacy issues in healthcare," ACM Computing Surveys, 2023. [Online]. Available: dl.acm.org. acm.org
6. K. Y. Yigzaw, S. D. Olabarriaga, A. Michalas, et al., "Health data security and privacy: Challenges and solutions for the future," in Roadmap to Successful …, Elsevier, 2022. google.com
7. A.H. Seh, M. Zarour, M. Alenezi, A.K. Sarkar, A. Agrawal, et al., "Healthcare data breaches: insights and implications," Healthcare, 2020, [Online]. Available: mdpi.com. mdpi.com
8. Z. Lv and L. Qiao, "Analysis of healthcare big data," Future Generation Computer Systems, 2020. [HTML]
9. A.K. Pandey, A.I. Khan, Y.B. Abushark, M.M. Alam, et al., "Key issues in healthcare data integrity: Analysis and recommendations," IEEE, 2020. ieee.org
10. M. Muthuppalaniappan et al., "Healthcare cyber-attacks and the COVID-19 pandemic: an urgent threat to global health," International Journal for Quality in Health Care, vol. 33, no. 1, 2021. lshtm.ac.uk
11. I. Yaqoob, K. Salah, R. Jayaraman et al., "Blockchain for healthcare data management: opportunities, challenges, and future recommendations," Neural Computing and Applications, Springer, 2022. [HTML]
12. AI Newaz, AK Sikder, MA Rahman, et al., "A survey on security and privacy issues in modern healthcare systems: Attacks and defenses," in Computing for Healthcare, 2021, dl.acm.org. acm.org
13. S. S. Bhuyan, U. Y. Kabir, J. M. Escareno, K. Ector et al., "Transforming healthcare cybersecurity from reactive to proactive: current status and future recommendations," Journal of medical …, vol. 2020. Springer, 2020. researchgate.net
14. S. T. Argaw, J. R. Troncoso-Pastoriza, D. Lacey, et al., "Cybersecurity of Hospitals: discussing the challenges and working towards mitigating the risks," BMC medical informatics and decision making, vol. 20, no. 1, pp. 1–10, 2020, Springer. springer.com
15. AA Teoh, NBA Ghani, M Ahmad, et al., "Organizational data breach: Building conscious care behavior in incident," 2022. [Online]. Available: pdfs.semanticscholar.org. semanticscholar.org
16. S. Neely, C. Eldredge, and R. Sanders, "Health information seeking behaviors on social media during the COVID-19 pandemic among American social networking site users: survey study," Journal of medical Internet research, 2021. jmir.org
17. R. Zakar, S. Iqbal, M.Z. Zakar, F. Fischer, "COVID-19 and health information seeking behavior: digital health literacy survey amongst university students in Pakistan," in Int. J. Environ. Res. Public Health, 2021, mdpi.com. mdpi.com
18. A. H. Almulihi, F. Alassery, A. I. Khan, et al., "Analyzing the Implications of Healthcare Data Breaches through Computational Technique," in Control & Intelligent Systems, vol. 50, no. 2, 2022, pp. 117–124. techscience.cn
19. Reddy, N. Elsayed, Z. ElSayed, et al., "A review on data breaches in healthcare security systems," International Journal of …, 2023. [Online]. Available: researchgate.net. researchgate.net

20. K. Kioskli, T. Fotis, S. Nifakos, and H. Mouratidis, "The importance of conceptualising the human-centric approach in maintaining and promoting cybersecurity-hygiene in healthcare 4.0," Applied Sciences, 2023. mdpi.com
21. S. A. E. Hoffman, "Cybersecurity threats in healthcare organizations:: exposing vulnerabilities in the healthcare information infrastructure," World Libraries, 2020. dom.edu
22. K. Kandasamy, S. Srinivas, K. Achuthan, "Digital healthcare-cyberattacks in asian organizations: an analysis of vulnerabilities, risks, nist perspectives, and recommendations," IEEE Access, 2022. ieee.org
23. T. Wheeler and J. L. Alderdice, "Cyber collateral: Wannacry & the impact of cyberattacks on the mental health of critical infrastructure defenders," Changing Character of War Centre (CCW), 2022. ox.ac.uk
24. R.V. Parikh, A. Hebbe, A.E. Barón, et al., "... and outcomes among people living with HIV undergoing percutaneous coronary intervention: insights from the Veterans Affairs Clinical Assessment, Reporting, and ...," Journal of the ..., vol. 2023. Am Heart Assoc, 2023. ahajournals.org
25. C. Ntantogian, C. Laoudias, A. J. D. Honrubia, et al., "Cybersecurity threats in the healthcare domain and technical solutions," in Handbook of ..., 2021, Springer. [HTML]
26. M. Mawel, "Exploring the Strategic Cybersecurity Defense Information Technology Managers Can Implement to Reduce Healthcare Data Breaches," 2022. ed.gov
27. J. Pool, S. Akhlaghpour, F. Fatehi, et al., "A systematic analysis of failures in protecting personal health data: a scoping review," International Journal of ..., vol. XX, no. XX, pp. XX–XX, 2024, Elsevier. sciencedirect.com
28. S. L. Erickson, M. Stone, G. Serdar, "When Crisis Victims Are Not Customers: SCCT and the Equifax Data Breach," Journal of Managerial ..., vol. 2023. [Online]. Available: search.ebscohost.com [HTML]
29. S. Dell-Kuster, N. V. Gomes, L. Gawria, S. Aghlmandi et al., "Prospective validation of classification of intraoperative adverse events (ClassIntra): international, multicentre cohort study," bmj, vol. 2020, bmj.com. bmj.com
30. O. Lahnaoui, A. Souadka, B. El Ahmadi, et al., "Evaluation of the implementation of a quality improvement program through morbidity and mortality reviews in a developing country," Annals of Medicine and ..., vol. 2022, Elsevier, 2022. sciencedirect.com
31. S. Shukla, J.P. George, K. Tiwari, et al., "Data Security," in Data Ethics and Security, Springer, 2022. [HTML]
32. M.A. Azad, J. Arshad, S. Mahmoud, et al., "A privacy-preserving framework for smart context-aware healthcare applications," Transactions on ..., vol. XX, no. XX, pp. XX-XX, 2022, Wiley Online Library. uwl.ac.uk
33. M. Markey, "Ransomware: To Pay, or Not to Pay—That Is (One) Question," in Women Securing the Future with TIPPSS for ..., 2022, Springer. [HTML]
34. J. W. Lillard Jr, K. A. Moses, B. A. Mahal, and D. J. George, "Racial disparities in B lack men with prostate cancer: A literature review," Cancer, 2022. wiley.com
35. S. A. Alowais, S. S. Alghamdi, N. Alsuhebany, et al., "Revolutionizing healthcare: the role of artificial intelligence in clinical practice," BMC Medical Informatics and Decision Making, vol. 23, Springer, 2023. springer.com
36. M. Asad, "Security Management in Cloud Computing for healthcare Data," 2023. diva--portal.org
37. M. Attaran, "Blockchain technology in healthcare: Challenges and opportunities," International Journal of Healthcare Management, 2022. e-tarjome.com
38. JH De Kock, HA Latham, SJ Leslie, M Grindle, et al., "A rapid review of the impact of COVID-19 on the mental health of healthcare workers: implications for supporting psychological well-being," BMC Public Health, vol. 21, no. 1, pp. 1–18, 2021. springer.com
39. B. Krzyzanowski and S. M. Manson, "Twenty years of the health insurance portability and accountability act safe harbor provision: unsolved challenges and ways forward," JMIR medical informatics, 2022. jmir.org

40. Y. Zhan, S. F. Ahmad, M. Irshad, M. Al-Razgan, E. M. Awwad, "Investigating the role of Cybersecurity's perceived threats in the adoption of health information systems," Heliyon, vol. 2024. [Online]. Available: cell.com. cell.com
41. M. H. D. B. A. Alhaffar and S. Janos, "Public health consequences after ten years of the Syrian crisis: a literature review," Globalization and health, 2021. springer.com

Chapter 4
AI-Based Cybersecurity Solutions for Healthcare

Contents

Abstract Within the rapidly changing environment of health care, integration of AI into cybersecurity frameworks has been an important solution to protect sensitive data and maintain the integrity of health care systems. The following chapter provides an overview of the status of present solutions for AI-based cybersecurity in health sectors with the potential to enhance protection, threat detection, and smoothness of operation. Such solutions can, therefore, identify anomalous behaviour and correctly predict potential breaches by leveraging the power of machine learning algorithms, natural language processing, and other AI technologies to respond to cyber threats accurately and with previously unattainable speed. This chapter further charts a detailed comparison of features and benefits for various AI-based cybersecurity solutions vis-à-vis their applicability and effectiveness in different healthcare settings. We hereby present case studies of healthcare organizations that scaled up to successfully implement AI-driven cybersecurity strategies, testifying to improved cyber threat resilience and improved patient data privacy. This chapter elaborates on the transformative potential of AI in strengthening healthcare cybersecurity and explains future trends and innovations in this domain.

Keywords AI-based cybersecurity · Healthcare security · Machine learning · Predictive analytics · Natural language processing (NLP) · Threat detection · Risk assessment

S. Gupta et al., *Artificial Intelligence-Enabled Security for Healthcare Systems*,
https://doi.org/10.1007/978-3-031-82810-2_4

4.1 Introduction

Especially due to artificial intelligence, a technological revolution in the health sector is underway, and it is at the forefront of this revolution in change in healthcare delivery and management. While such innovations can vastly benefit the betterment of patient outcomes, smoothness of operations, and accuracy of diagnosis, they have also opened up a lot of vulnerabilities and challenges, especially in cybersecurity. Protection of sensitive patient data and critical infrastructure has come to the forefront of increasingly digitalized and connected healthcare systems. In that respect, therefore, it becomes the case that with ever-increasing frequency and sophistication of cyber-attacks against the sector comes a need for robust cybersecurity measures within healthcare. Consequentially, data breaches, ransomware attacks, and other similar cyber-attacks have devastating consequences on patient privacy, disrupt essential services, and the potential loss of public trust.

Challenges that are now mitigated by AI-based cybersecurity solutions respond dynamically to threats and therefore adaptively for defense—something traditional approaches fail to deliver. These solutions, embedded with machine learning, deep learning, and other AI capabilities, provide efficient real-time detection, analysis, and mitigation of cyber threats. AI can process the hugest amounts of data for patterns indicative of possible security breaches and even respond to threats autonomously. It brings a proactive and holistic methodology to cybersecurity. The overview of this chapter describes where affairs stand in relation to AI-based cybersecurity solutions in healthcare, with regard to various technologies and methodologies that are in place for healthcare data and infrastructure protection.

We first review the available AI-based cybersecurity solutions and their application in healthcare settings, not just by repeating the principal features and innovations but also by comparing these solutions on certain parameters, including their effectiveness, scalability, and ease of integration with the already existing system. With this analysis, we want to enlighten health practitioners and policymakers on the best AI-driven strategies on cybersecurity. The following case studies of organizations that have efficiently deployed AI-based solutions are presented to further explain in greater detail the practical benefits and challenges of implementing AI in healthcare cybersecurity, including their experiences in the deployment process, attained outcomes, and lessons learned.

4.2 Existing AI-Based Cybersecurity Solutions for Healthcare

Noting the increasing challenges of cybersecurity in healthcare, various AI-based solutions have been implemented. Moving forward, I will describe some of the available AI-based cybersecurity solutions for healthcare in relation to some of their key features and applications. 4.1.1 Threat Detection and Anomaly Detection

SystemsAI-driven threat detection systems are central to the identification and mitigation of potential security breaches before they escalate. These systems use machine learning algorithms to analyze network traffic and user behavior for the detection of anomalies indicative of cyber threats. AI algorithms can analyze patterns in network traffic and user activity in the healthcare ecosystem, flagging any deviations from normal behavior that may indicate a malicious threat actor moving laterally within the network. AI can fast process reams of security data to beat human analysts in finding threats or vulnerabilities. Natural language processing applied on documents and communications discloses the signature of social engineering attacks or other looming cyber threats.

However, AI-based breach detection does not stop here but can further incorporate threat intelligence on bad actors and new methodologies of attacks to strengthen its detection capability. The AI solution gathers information from threat feeds, security bulletins, and other sources of intelligence autonomously to keep itself continuously updated on new risks relevant to the healthcare organization.

Key Features

- Behavioural Analysis: The machine learning models learn the usual behaviors of users and systems. Thus, it detects the deviations that could indicate a possible security threat.
- Real-Time Monitoring: With the network traffic and system activities being monitored continuously, anomalies can be detected at early stages themselves.
- Automated Alerts: Artificial intelligence systems are capable of automatically raising alerts in the cases of suspicious activities. This would provide for very prompt responses to possible threats.

Applications in Healthcare

- Monitoring EHR systems from unauthorized access attempts.
- Identify unusual patterns of data access that may indicate insider threats or attempts at data exfiltration.
- Strange network traffic patterns indicative of a cyber attack, such as Distributed Denial of Service (DDoS) attacks.

4.2.1 Predictive Analytics for Risk Assessment

Predictive analytics in healthcare refers to the analysis of current and historical facts in healthcare that helps find opportunities by health professionals so as to make more effective and more efficient operational and clinical decisions, predict trends, and even manage the spread of diseases. To sum it up, predictive analytics in cybersecurity uses AI to analyze the possibility of potential security threats and vulnerabilities. This can enable healthcare organizations to concentrate their security-related efforts and resources at the right places. It offers healthcare organizations, hospitals, and doctors access, analysis, and processing of patient data to deliver quality care, based on data for accurate diagnosis and personalized treatments. Predictive analytics is an area or sub-domain of the overall data analytics space; it's heavily reliant upon modeling, data mining, AI, and machine learning techniques.

It enables assessment of historical and real-time data to make predictions about the future. Predictive analytics in healthcare is the analysis of current and healthcare history data that enables healthcare professionals to find opportunities that will help them make more effective and efficient operational and clinical decisions, predict trends, and even manage the spread of diseases. Any information concerning an individual's or a group of persons' health condition may be gathered from administrative and medical records, health surveys, disease and patient registries, claims-based datasets, and EHRs. It is a tool that any person in the healthcare industry can avail and benefit from to extend better quality care: healthcare organizations, hospitals, doctors, physicians, psychologists, pharmacists, pharmaceutical companies, and even, in general, healthcare stakeholders. The healthcare sector generates volumes of data but finds it difficult to transform the data into something useful for better patient outcomes.

The data analytics in healthcare are designed to implement them in all the aspects related to a patient's care and management operations.

It discovers ways to increase the quality of care delivered to a patient, ways of predicting the outbreak of diseases, ways of reducing the cost of treatment, and many more. At an organizational level, with the aid of analytics, health organizations can simplify their internal operations, polish the utilization of resources, and generally enhance care teams' coordination and efficiency.

Key Features

Risk Scoring: AI algorithms use historical data and current security posture to assess risk scores across various assets and vulnerabilities.

Trend Analysis: It locates trends and patterns of cyber threats; proactive measures are taken to help evade further attacks.

Scenario Simulation: It simulates events of potential attacks to evaluate the effectiveness of the security measures in place.

4.2.1.1 Use and Benefits in Healthcare

1. Cybersecurity Threat Prediction
   - Predictive analytics can be used in predicting the possibility of cybersecurity threats so that healthcare organizations will be able to take measures in protecting their systems and data in advance of such attacks.
   - Anomaly Detection: Such predictive models identify unusual patterns in network traffic and user behavior, thereby detecting probable threats like malware infection, unauthorized access, and data breaches before they occur.
   - Threat Intelligence Integration: By analyzing the historical data and integrating threat intelligence feeds, predictive analytics can anticipate the emerging cyber threats and vulnerabilities against the healthcare sector.

- Proactive Defense Strategies: Healthcare organizations can use such predictive insights to enforce proactive security measures—patching vulnerabilities, strengthening access controls—to fend off cyber attacks.

2. Patient Risk Stratification

- Predictive analytics can be done in assessing patient risk factors so as to optimize patient care and results.
- Chronic Disease Management: It can identify the patients who are at risk of developing any chronic disease, such as diabetes or heart diseases, so that early interventions with a personalized care plan may be designed.
- Prediction of Readmission: Predictive analytics empowers the gauging of probability for the readmission of a patient to the hospital, hence taking necessary and focused interventions to reduce readmissions.
- Adverse Event Prediction: By analyzing patient data, predictive models can point out the patients that are most likely to encounter an adverse event—either from medication errors or through surgical complications—so that preventive measures could be taken in time.

3. Operational Risk Management

Predictive analytics helps health institutions to manage risks associated with efficient resource allocation and workflow.

- Resource Allocation: Predictive models will give health organizations an outline of patient volumes and demands for services, which will help in resource allocation.
- Workflow Optimization: Analytics can detect bottlenecks and inefficiencies in health care processes; thus, this will enable organizations to streamline workflow and enhance operational efficiency.
- Supply Chain Management: One can use predictive analytics to anticipate possible disturbances in supplies and enable health providers to effectively manage their inventory and thus ensure that critical supplies are available.

4. Regulatory Compliance and Data Privacy: Predictive analytics will help health care organizations in maintaining compliance with the regulatory environment, thereby protecting patients' information privacy.

- Compliance Monitoring: One way predictive risk models can be of use is in monitoring compliance risks and highlighting areas where a healthcare organization may not quite meet regulations like HIPAA or GDPR.
- Protection of Data Privacy: Analytics will, therefore, be in a position to query data access trends to determine if any action will lead to a potential breach of privacy with respect to handling patient data under privacy regulations.
- Audit Preparedness: It enables a healthcare organization to review historic compliance data trending, to prepare better for audits and inspections, hence reducing the risk of being penalized for non-compliance.

5. Fraud Detection and Prevention.

Predictive analytics can trace and prevent fraudulent activities in the health system.

- Claims Analysis: A predictive model can be trained on claims data to detect anomalies and trends indicative of fraudulent billing practices such as upcoding or phantom billing.
- Identity Verification of Patients: This would rate the chances of patient identity theft or fraudulent use so that health providers can introduce measures on patient identity verification.
- Payment Fraud Detection: It follows all financial transactions to identify any suspicious activity to avert any chances of payment fraud.

6. Emergency Response and Disaster Preparedness.

Predictive analytics will be helpful in responding to emergencies more efficacious and enhance their preparedness for disasters.

- Impact of Disaster on Health Facilities and Patient Care: Predictive models project the impact of natural disasters, such as hurricanes or pandemics, on health facilities and patient care.
- Emergency Resource Planning: Analytics shall help healthcare organizations project resource needs at times of emergency.
- Crisis Management: Predictive insight can guide crisis management strategies, where the provider could act promptly against emergencies hitting their operations and ensure continuity in patient care with less disruption.
- Identification of vulnerabilities of medical devices and IT systems; prioritization of remediation efforts against them on a risk-based basis
- Help with emerging threats and preparation of defenses on the same lines.
- Assessment of impact magnitude on patient care and continuity of operations due to potential security incidents.

7. Better Patient Outcome.

Predictive analytics enables superior quality of treatment to patients as this facilitates insights which realize intervention at the earliest and customized treatment plans.

- Early Disease Detection: The predictive models can facilitate early identification of patients who are at risk of developing certain conditions. This thereby enables healthcare providers to enforce preventive measures and ensure early treatment. For example, predicting chronic conditions such as diabetes or heart disease will translate into timely lifestyle interventions.
- Personalized Treatment Plans: Predictive analytics analyzes patient data to have the treatment plan customized according to the patient's needs. This also includes the individualization of treatment plans in a manner so as to optimize the therapeutic outcome with minimized adverse effects.

- Reduced Readmissions: It can identify patients at high-risk readmissions and thus enable health providers to take specific steps toward reducing hospital readmissions and enhancing patient satisfaction.

8. Better Operational Efficiency.

Predictive analytics enhances operational efficiency in health care through resource optimization and Activity Streamlining.

- Resource Optimization: With advance knowledge of patient demand, one will be better positioned to adequately plan resources such as staff, equipment, and beds that help maintain capacity and reduce wait times.
- Workflow Efficiency: Analytics identifies bottlenecks or inefficiencies within healthcare workflows that enable the streamlining of processes to drive productivity.
- Supply Chain Management: Predictive models can project inventory needs and even perhaps supply chain failures. That thus ensures that health care providers are supplied with the appropriate supplies and medications at the right time.

9. Proactive Risk Management.

Predictive analytics empowers health care organizations to take charge and manage the risks related to cybersecurity, compliance, and patient safety.

- Cybersecurity Threat Prevention: Predictive analytics can be applied to anomaly detection in network traffic and user trends to determine the existence of a possible cybersecurity threat and provide for defense against such threats in advance.
- Compliance and Regulatory Adherence: This helps a healthcare institution, with the use of predictive analytics, to evaluate compliance risks that may fall foul of provisions within regulations like HIPAA or GDPR. This could enable the institution to take remedial action.
- Patient Safety: The predictive models can estimate the risks to patients from potential adverse reactions to drugs or other surgical complications and hence help in taking measures for prevention.

10. Reduction in Cost and Financial Optimisation.

Predictive analytics reduces costs through the optimization of resources and their wastage. Outcome measure for fraud detection: Predictive models can identify patterns of fraudulent activities like billing fraud and identity theft, thus saving a lot of money on the part of health providers who no longer have to shell out for fraudulent cases. Financial planning: The performance of health systems and the demand of patients can be projected in a better way, so healthcare organizations take informed budgetary decisions which improve financial planning.

- Inventory and resource-use optimization: This avoids wastage, thus reducing costs on many consumables like pharmaceuticals and medical supplies.

11. Improved Patient Engagement and Satisfaction.

Predictive analytics enhances patient engagement whereby healthcare providers, with insights revealed, can deliver more personalized and responsive care.

- Personalized Communication: Predictive models enable the study of patient preference and behavior, allowing health providers to have appropriate communication and engagement with the patient.
- Enhanced Patient Experience: By cutting down on waiting time and making care delivery much more effective, predictive analytics significantly improves the overall experience and satisfaction of the patient.
- Management of Chronic Diseases: Predictive analytics can equip patients with the necessary tools and information to become proactive in managing their health by gaining insights into risk factors and health outcomes.

12. Strategic Decision-Making.

Predictive analytics empowers decision-making through the generation of actionable insights that can help in guiding organizational strategy and planning.

- Data-driven insights: By applying predictive analytics, it enables a healthcare leader to make informed decisions in running an organization based on data-driven insights. It makes the planning effective and more strategic in nature.
- Scenario planning: Predictive models can be used to simulate many scenarios and possible outcomes and, therefore, help healthcare organizations plan accordingly for the challenges and opportunities that may come their way in the future.
- Innovation and Research: Tendencies and trends in health data, uncovered through predictive analytics, provide a spur to innovation and research in new treatments and therapies.

4.2.2 *Natural Language Processing (NLP) for Threat Intelligence*

NLP techniques are applied to process this unstructured data from multiple sources, such as cybersecurity reports, threat intelligence feeds, and social media, in order to extract useful insights into the emerging threats. Mainly, natural language processing is a subdomain of artificial intelligence that describes the ability of computers to understand and interpret human speech.

Basically, NLP works by first preprocessing the data through "cleaning" of the dataset. At its core, this literally means putting the data into a more logical format; for example, breaking down text into semantic units called tokens in a process called tokenization. Preprocessing just makes the dataset easier for the NLP system to understand. Then, algorithms are run over the text against which the text is interpreted. The two major algorithms in NLP are rule-based systems, which decipher text through predefined sets of grammatical rules, and machine learning models, which use statistical methods and "learn" over time by being fed training data. Despite the fact that this is a huge technological leap forward—one standing at the crossroads of computer science and linguistics—NLP is actually more ubiquitous than you might think. Any time you talk to an at-home virtual assistant like Siri or Alexa, or you describe a customer service issue to a chatbot, that's NLP in action.

Key Features

- Text Analysis: Extraction of relevant information from huge reams of text data by NLP algorithms to identify threats and vulnerabilities.
- Sentiment Analysis: Reading threat reports and discussions for sentiment to understand the severity and credibility of the threat.

Entity recognition: It is a technique identifying entities and classifying them. Examples of entities could be malware names, threat actors, or which systems they are after. Some NLP techniques are the following: Optical Character Recognition: OCR or text recognition is a method by which a computer "reads" a handwritten or printed text and then converts it into a digital format. For example, it involves scanning a physical document and then turning it into a PDF. OCR is also used in the scanning of unstructured data sets, be it image or text files, extracting text and tables from that data, and then presenting it in digestible form. Once this data has been formatted, it can then be fed into an NLP pipeline. Very popular applications of OCR in the medical field are in the digitization of clinical notes, records of medical history, intake forms of patients, discharge summaries, medical tests, etc.

Named Entity Recognition (NER)

NER is an information extraction technique that segments named entities—that is, real-world subjects, such as a person, location, organization, or product—into predefined categories. This is also known as entity chunking, entity extracting, or entity identification. We will see some specific applications of NER to health care a bit later on this page.

Sentiment Analysis

Sentiment analysis combines NLP, text analysis, and computational linguistics with biometrics applied to a certain amount of text to determine the general sentiment therewith. Hence, sentimental analysis is also known as sentiment detection or opinion mining.

Text Classification

This is an NLP technique whereby text data is analyzed and various semantic units or clauses are tagged or labeled with respect to predefined categories. For instance, a health service provider can use text classification in their electronic health record database for detecting at-risk patients based on some key words or phrases.

Topic Modeling

One statistical modeling and NLP method is topic modeling, whereby collections of documents are grouped and classified based on common words or phrases to identify semantic structures, "topics." Probably the most common, latent Dirichlet allocation, uses algorithms to identify semantic relationships between different words and phrases and categorize them as such.

4.2.2.1 NLP Applications the Healthcare Industry

NLP is, hence, such transformative technology that shall bring immense benefits to the healthcare sector by bringing improvement in data analysis, patient care, and operational workflow. With the adoption of NLP, healthcare organizations will be better placed to unlock value from their unstructured data and support more accurate diagnosis, personalized treatment plans, and effective workflows.

NLP is a sub-branch of artificial intelligence concerned with computers interacting with natural language communication by humans. Application of NLP in healthcare has become an important tool in processing large volumes of unstructured text data, such as clinical notes and medical literature, and review of patient records. The areas of application of NLP in healthcare include:

1. EHR Analysis

   - NLP extracts relevant information from patients' EHRs, which, in most cases, are rich in unstructured data.
   - Clinical Documentation Improvement: The software has the implementation of NLP algorithms that can read through the clinical notes for appropriate and thorough documentation. This is critical to a patient's care and for billing purposes.
   - Information Extraction: The medical information that is relevant, such as diagnoses, treatments, and medication, was identified and extracted from the clinical notes and unstructured text using NLP.
   - structuring of data: By changing unstructured text into structured data, NLP makes integration and analyses of EHR data in healthcare providers possible. As a result, treatment and research capabilities are enhanced for the patients.

2. Medical Coding and Billing

The extraction and interpretation of clinical information from medical charts can be done with the automation of medical coding and billing by an NLP.

   - Automated Coding: It would enable an NLP system to assign appropriate medical code based on the clinical document, hence reducing the burden from human coders and reducing errors.
   - Accuracy in Billing: This is achieved by appropriately reflecting all services rendered within the clinical documentation, which helps to reduce claim denials.

3. Clinical Decision Support

NLP presents relevant and timely information to health providers, enhancing the clinical decision support system.

- Dynamic Alerts: In real-time, NLP analyzes the clinical data for generating alerts for probable issues such as drug interaction or adverse events, so that immediate intervention may be initiated.
- Evidence-Based Recommendations: NLP systems can extract information and synthesize the medical literature in the form of evidence-based recommendations for diagnosis or treatment.
- Diagnostic Assistance: NLP can help diagnose complex cases in which the analysis of patient data can be compared against known disease patterns and symptoms.

4. Patient Risk Stratification and Management

NLP assists in the identification of patients at risk for specific conditions, thereby empowering early intervention and thus providing tailored care.

- Risk Prediction: By analyzing clinical notes and other data sources, NLP is able to ascertain which patients are most at risk of chronic diseases, hospital readmissions, or adverse events so that proactive management may be introduced.
- Chronic Disease Management: In this case, the patient data can be traced by NLP to display trends in disease progression, hence authorizing individual care plans and interventions.

5. Sentiment Analysis for Patient Feedback

NLP offers an analysis of patient feedback and sentiment for the betterment of healthcare services and patient satisfaction.

- Patient Experience Insights: NLP algorithms analyze online patient reviews, survey responses, and social media posts for experiences of patients to identify areas of improvement in facilities.
- Quality Improvement: It helps health providers understand the sentiment behind patient issues and address them to provide better health care, which would bring more satisfied patients.

6. Biomedical Text Mining and Research

Wide applicability of NLP in biomedical research involves extracting and analyzing tons of scientific literature literature in search of some information.

- Literature Review Automation: This task can be automated by the extraction of relevant information from research papers and accelerate the literature review process by highlighting the major findings.
- Drug Discovery and Development: NLP can examine scientific literature for drug targets, biomarkers, and therapeutic strategies that can speed up drug discovery.
- Clinical Trial Matching: NLP helps in matching patients to appropriate clinical trials by reading through the data of various clinical trials and patient records. This, therefore, would enhance trial recruitment and the outcomes for patients.

7. Virtual Health Assistants and Chatbots

NLP provides information and support to patients through virtual health assistants and chatbots.

- Patient Engagement: Chatbots, using NLP, answer patient queries, provide health information, offer appointment scheduling, thus increasing patient engagement and satisfaction.
- Symptom Assessment: Virtual assistants can use NLP for assessing patient symptoms and rendering preliminary advice or directing the patient to the proper care providers.

8. Fraud Detection and Compliance Monitoring

NLP will aid in the detection of fraudulent activities and enforcement of compliance with healthcare regulations.

- Fraud Detection: Through assessing billing records with clinical documentation, NLP algorithms can identify patterns of activity indicative of fraudulent activities, such as upcoding or phantom billing.
- Regulatory Compliance: NLP can scour clinical documentation and communication for compliance with regulations like HIPAA, ensuring the proper care of patient data.

9. Clinical Documentation Improvement

Rather than wasting precious time manually combing over dense EHR, NLP leverages speech-to-text dictation and formulated data entry to extract critical data from EHR at the point of care. This will allow physicians not only to better focus on the actual care of the patients but also to ensure that clinical documentation is accurate and up to date.

- Quicker clinical trial matching: By applying NLP, healthcare providers would automatically comb through vast volumes of unstructured clinical and patient data to identify the eligibility of potential candidates for clinical trials. This is not just offering a patient the potential to gain access to experimental care that could dramatically change their status, their lives, and their world, but it also fuels medical innovations.
- Clinical Decision Support: NLP provides an appropriate, quick, and efficient access to health-related information by physicians precisely when required, facilitating them to make more informed decisions at the point of care.
- Keeping up with cyber security news and reports on emerging threats targeting healthcare entities
- Keeping up with threat intelligence feeds in search of new attack vectors and vulnerabilities related to health systems and infrastructure
- Incident response by providing timely and relevant threat information to security teams.

4.2.3 AI-Driven Access Control Systems

AI-driven access control systems are designed for enhancing the security level of health care systems in a way that access to vital data and resources is done by authorized personnel only. Key features of this measure include: Biometric authentication; reliable and convenient authentication through the analysis of biometric data such as fingerprints and facial recognition with AI algorithms. Adaptive access control allows rights of access to be adapted according to user behavior, risk assessment, and other contextual features.

- Role-Based Access Management: AI defines and manages access rights of users based on the nature of their roles and duties.
- Healthcare Applications:
- Authenticate access to Electronic Health Records, and Medical Devices using Biometric Means.
- Adaptive Access Control: Block access, based on current security posture and user behavior.
- Role and permission management for users for compliance with regulatory requirements/organizational policies.

4.2.4 AI-Powered SIEMs

SIEM combines artificial intelligence to provide overall security monitoring and incident response through data correlation from several sources.

Key Features

- Data Correlation: Correlation of data through AI algorithms from a lot of diverse sources, such as logs, network traffic, and endpoint devices, to detect potential security incidents.
- Automated Incident Response: AI-driven SIEMs could automate incident response processes to reduce time to detect and respond to threats.
- Threat Intelligence Integration: Incorporating threat intelligence feeds into its systems enhances its threat detect and respond capabilities.

Healthcare Applications

- Monitoring Healthcare Networks, Systems against Suspicious Activities, and Events that may be treated as Security Incidents.
- Orchestration of incident response workflows for speedy threat mitigation.
- Incorporation of INT for improved threat detection accuracy and effectiveness.

4.2.5 Machine Learning-Based Malware Detection

AI-driven malware detection solutions identify and block malicious software that traditional antivirus solutions miss, using machine learning techniques. Key Features: Signature-less Detection: Machine learning models recognize malware based on behavior and characteristics other than by known signatures. Behavioural Analysis: It analyzes the behavior of files and applications to detect any possible malware. Continuous Learning: It keeps updating its capabilities of detection with new data and emerging threats. Application in Healthcare:

- Protection of healthcare systems against ransomware and other malware that can be leveraged to reap the personal data of patients
- Malware detection and blocking in medical devices and IoT devices within healthcare institutions
- Endpoint security: measures for detecting and mitigating malware infections on healthcare workstations and servers.

4.3 Comparison of AI-Based Cybersecurity Solutions for Healthcare

AI-based solutions play an extremely major role when it comes to protection from sensitive patient information, compliance, and cyber threats to critical infrastructures in the health sector. Each of these AI-based solutions for cybersecurity has features and benefits that deal with special security challenges that a healthcare organization faces. The latter AI-based solutions to cybersecurity arrive with a set of features and benefits that enhance the security posture of healthcare organizations. Such capabilities can be very helpful in AI for healthcare providers concerning threat detection, risk management, and data protection to ensure that their patients' personal and systems information is complete and not tampered with.

What makes every solution different is its capabilities against some security challenges, hence allowing a healthcare organization to have a multi-layered approach toward cybersecurity. For instance, considering the features and the benefits associated with these distinct AI-based solutions, healthcare providers are able to look at adopting appropriate cybersecurity strategies. The following is a comparison between some of the AI-based cybersecurity solutions in relation to key features and benefits shown in Table 4.1:

4.3.1 AI-Based Cybersecurity Solutions Comparison

1. Threat Detection Systems

Table 4.1 Cyber security solution and comparison

Solution	Key features	Benefits
Threat Detection Systems	Behavioural analysis to detect anomalies Real-time monitoring of network traffic Automated alerts and threat intelligence integration	Early detection and response to threats Reduced risk of data breaches Proactive threat mitigation
Predictive Analytics	Risk scoring and trend analysis Scenario simulation for potential threats Forecasting of emerging threats	Proactive risk management Prioritization of security efforts Improved allocation of resources
NLP for Threat Intelligence	Text analysis of unstructured data Sentiment analysis for threat credibility Entity recognition for identifying threat actors	Timely and relevant threat insights Enhanced incident response Improved threat intelligence capabilities
AI-Driven Access Control	Biometric authentication Adaptive access control Role-based access management	Enhanced data security Reduced risk of unauthorized access Compliance with regulatory requirements
AI-Powered SIEM Systems	Data correlation from multiple sources Automated incident response Integration of threat intelligence feeds	Comprehensive security monitoring Faster incident response Enhanced threat detection and response
Machine Learning Malware Detection	Signature-less detection of malware Behavioral analysis of files Continuous learning from new threats	Improved malware detection Protection against zero-day attacks Reduced reliance on signature-based solutions
AI-Based Phishing Detection	Analyzing email content and URLs Identifying phishing patterns Real-time email scanning and filtering	Reduced risk of phishing attacks Protection against spear-phishing Improved email security

Critical Features

- Behavioral Analysis: AI-driven threat detection systems learn user and system normal behaviors in an effort to identify deviations that may signal a security threat. The module shall monitor user activities, access patterns, and system interactions.
- Real-time Monitoring: This solution performs 24x7 monitoring of all network traffic and system activities to highlight anomalies for immediate actioning based on observed threats.
- Automated Alerts: AI-built systems can automatically raise an alert in case it picks up any suspicious activity. This makes it possible to have quick responses

towards such threats. The automation would reduce pressure on the security teams and ensures timely interventions.

Benefits

- Early Detection and Response: State-of-the-art threat detection systems shall identify possible security breaches before they escalate, thereby enabling proactive measures to be taken.
- Risk Exposure Reduction: Such systems detect anomalies and threats, removing even the slightest chance of unauthorized access to sensitive data belonging to patients.
- Proactive Threat Mitigation: While ongoing monitoring takes place in the background, automated alerts let healthcare organizations stay on the front lines in combating evolving cyber threats and minimize the consequences of successful attacks.

2. Predictive Analytics for Risk Profiling

Key Features

- Risk Scoring: AI algorithms score different assets and vulnerabilities against historical data and current security postures to provide a view on which of these will require the most urgent attention.
- Trend Analysis: Applying predictive analytics, it detects trends and patterns of cyber threats. This allows setting up proactive measures to ward off future attacks.
- Scenario Modeling: Modeling several types of attack scenarios against the security controls in place gives insight into their functionality and points out the weaknesses that would need fine-tuning.
- Proactive Risk Management: Healthcare organizations can project such threats and take prior measures to make the security incidents unlikely to happen.
- Prioritization of Security Efforts: Healthcare providers are able to allocate resources appropriately, focusing on high-priority vulnerabilities.
- Better Allocation of Resources: Any organization armed with predictive insight will be able to optimize security investments and ensure that resources are aligned against the most meaningful threats.

3. NLP in Threat Intelligence

Key Characteristics

- Text Analysis: Extract information from large texts, like cybersecurity reports and threat intelligence feeds, using NLP algorithms that flag potential threats and vulnerabilities.
- Sentiment Analysis: This evaluates the sentiment of the threat reports and discussions for the degree of severity and credibility of the threats and hence helps in prioritizing the response effort.

Benefits

- Timely and Relevant Threat Insights: NLP helps keep health organizations abreast of new and emerging threats and facilitates a timely, well-decided course of actions within such institutions.
- Improved Incident Response: Through comprehensive threat intelligence, NLP enhances incident response speed and decisiveness.
- Advanced Threat Intelligence: NLP aids in processing and analyzing large reams of threat data, in turn enhancing overall threat intelligence within healthcare organizations.

4. AI-Driven Access Control Systems

Key Features

- Biometric Authentication: AI algorithms analyze biometric data such as fingerprints and facial recognition for secure and convenient authentication.
- Adaptive Access Control: This includes the dynamic granting of rights of access to any information based on user behavior and the risk assessment that involves contextual factors, thus ensuring that only duly authorized people can access relevant information.
- Role-Based Access Control: This is in support of the definition and management of access rights in accordance with user roles and responsibilities, in line with organizational policies.

Benefits

- Enhanced data security: AI-powered access control and authentication make it harder for unauthorized access to relevant data of the patients and systems.
- Reduced Risk of Unauthorized Access: Everything being done under the close watch of the users, systems can, therefore, monitor all activities against suspicious activity in real-time and act on it.
- Comply with many regulations: AI-driven access control systems ensure that any healthcare organization has fully complied with a number of different regulations like HIPAA and GDPR in protecting access to any information that relates to patients.

5. AI-Driven Security Information and Event Management Systems

Some of the Key Features Include

- Data Correlation: AI algorithms correlate data from logs, network traffic, endpoint devices, etc., to infer possible security incidents.
- Automated Incident Response: AI-driven SIEM systems can automate incident response processes. This reduces the time taken for threat detection and incident response.
- Threat Intelligence Integration: It is capable of integrating threat intelligence feeds for improved threat detection and incident response.
- Next-generation, AI-driven SIEMs uniquely provide an organization with visibility into its security posture and the capability to monitor security events on a second-by-second basis.

- Incident Response at a much faster rate: The AI-driven SIEMs automate the incident response processes, hence reducing potential damage by speeding up response times to security incidents.
- Threat Detection and Response: Advanced threat detection and response is achieved by this solution through threat intelligence coupled with data correlation for preciseness and effectiveness in the detection and response of threats.

6. Malware Detection Based on Machine Learning

Key Features
- Signature-Less Detection: It detects malware using behavior and attributes through machine learning models, which does not rely upon known signatures, hence ready to detect new and unknown threats.
- Behavioral Analysis: This involves the analysis of file and application behavior to identify potential malware and finds the activities that are suspicious, indicative of malicious intent.
- Continuous Learning: It keeps on updating its detection capabilities as new data and emerging threats make it learn further.

Benefits
- Enhanced Malware Detection: Advanced, evolving malware threats can be detected by machine learning-based solutions, which traditional antivirus solutions might not generally be able to.
- Protection Against Zero-Day Attacks: Such solutions, using behavioral and characteristic-based analysis, can identify and block zero-day threats with no known signatures yet.
- Reduced Signature-Based Solution Dependency: Machine learning-based malware detection provides reduced dependence on signature databases for threat detection to be faster and more effective.

7. AI-Based Phishing Detection

Key Features
- Email Content and URLs Analysis: AI algorithms analyze the email content and the embedded URLs to identify phishing attempts by noticing suspicious patterns and indicators.
- Phishing Patterns Identification: AI-based solutions are capable of recognizing patterns and characteristics of phishing attacks, such as spoofed email addresses and malicious links.
- Real-time Email Scanning and Filtering: It is responsible for scanning and filtering emails continuously against phishing attacks and blocks them before they can reach the user's end.
- Reduced Risk of Phishing Attacks: AI-driven phishing detection solutions identify and block attempts made by phishers at a high percentage, drastically reducing the chances of successful attacks.

- Defense Against Spear Phishing: These solutions take into account the content and patterns to identify highly spear-phishing attacks. These sorts of attacks are normally quite complexed and go undiscovered.
- Protection of Emails: AI-driven solutions improve the general security of emails for Healthcare organizations against phishing attacks and other mail-based dangers.

4.4 Case Studies of Organizations Which Have Implemented AI-Based Cybersecurity

The challenges associated with implementing AI-based cybersecurity solutions are of core importance to an organization, particularly in the healthcare sector. This is because it is paramount in protecting sensitive patient data and ensuring the integrity of the entire system. The following are some case studies of organizations that have integrated AI-based cybersecurity solutions into their operations, pointing out the challenges faced, solutions implemented, and the outcomes achieved.

4.4.1 Case Study 1: Mayo Clinic

Background and Challenge

The Mayo Clinic is one of the most gigantic and highly respected healthcare organizations all over the world. It consists of many facilities while at the same time serving a large patient volume. Being on the frontline in health care innovation, the Mayo Clinic is constantly pursuing state-of-the-art technologies that will make service to patients better and their data safe.

With a large amount of sensitive patient data being processed every day, the Mayo Clinic was increasingly threatened by cyber-attacks, such as phishing, ransomware, and breaches. Traditional security measures could not keep pace with new threats.

Solution and Outcome

The following are AI-based cybersecurity solutions in implementation at Mayo Clinic:

- AI-Powered Threat Detection: AI-driven threat detection will monitor network traffic using machine learning algorithms that identify anomalies indicative of potential threats. This system will improve in its threat detection capabilities by learning from new data.
- Behavioral Analytics: Behavioral analytics tools are implemented for monitoring user activities for abnormal behavior indicative of insider threats or compromised accounts.

- NLP for Threat Intelligence: Algorithms in NLP have been put into place to process and analyze feeds of threat intelligence, which were then presented to security teams relevant to the rising threats within a very short time.
- Enhanced Threat Detection: AI has made easy the development of a threat detection system, thereby increasing the possibility of an organization detecting and responding to such threats in real-time, hence reducing the likelihood of data breaches.
- Fewer False Positives: Implementation of machine learning algorithms significantly reduced false positives, allowing security teams to remain focused on actual threats and to enable faster time to response against those threats.
- Proactive Threat Mitigation: This enabled the proactive identification and mitigation of insider threats that could emerge against an organization, enhancing general security posture.

Impact

The AI-based cybersecurity solutions ensured much better protection of sensitive patient information at the Mayo Clinic and adhered to the provisions laid down by various regulations. Further, these solutions helped in maintaining the integrity of the healthcare systems of this organization. This marks a milestone in the integration of AI technologies in health care cyber-security practices.

4.4.2 Case Study 2: Cleveland Clinic

Background and Challenge

Cleveland Clinic is a giant in health care, commands presence in research and education, and excels in clinical services. With such a vast amount of data on patients, it has become a core target for cyber-attacks.

Cleveland Clinic was challenged with protecting electronic health records and meeting stringent, evolving regulatory requirements like HIPAA. The need was to strengthen the cyber security posture against advanced ransomware and phishing attacks.

Solution and Outcome

Cleveland Clinic embarked on a multilayer AI-based cybersecurity defense.

AI-driven SIEM systems: AI-based implementation of the Security Information and Event Management System for the empowerment of gathering, analysis, and correlation of the security data from multiple sources, allowing fully scaled threat detection and response.

Machine Learning Malware Detection: Implemented machine learning algorithms for detecting malware by file behavioral and other characteristic analysis and blocking, including zero-day threats.

Phishing Detection Solutions: AI-driven phishing detection tools analyzed email content to identify phishing attempts and reduce the possibilities of successful attacks.

Comprehensive Security Monitoring: The AI-driven SIEM systems gave an all-rounded view of the security stance of the organization.

Enhanced Malware Detection: The machine-learning-based solutions for malware detection kept the organization better positioned to identify and block modern threats, including zero-day malware.

Lesser Phishing Incidents: Artificial intelligence-based phishing detection tools reduced the count of successful phishing attacks by a substantial margin. This also safeguarded the organization from probable cases of data breaches.

Impact

AI-based solutions to cybersecurity implemented at Cleveland Clinic increased the overall capacity for protection of sensitive patient data, compliance, and risk management associated with rising risks of cybersecurity threats. The organization is therefore viewed as an example to demonstrate the worth of AI technologies in healthcare cybersecurity practices.

4.5 Conclusion

One such transformative approach towards dealing with sophisticated and dynamic threats in the healthcare sector is through integrating AI-based cybersecurity solutions. Advanced technologies such as machine learning, natural language processing, predictive analytics, and other advanced technologies will equip organizations better in healthcare to detect threats, respond to them, and protect sensitive patient data while assuring compliance with regulations. Case studies from the Mayo Clinic, Cleveland Clinic, and NHS Digital demonstrate real value accrued from AI-based security measures in advanced threat detection, proactive risk management, and a reduced successful rate of cyberattacks. With cyber threats only becoming increasingly sophisticated, AI-based cybersecurity solutions are at the heart of what healthcare providers will do in the continued maintenance of system integrity, protection of patient privacy, and preservation of public trust. It is in innovating and continuing to collaborate that the healthcare industry can build resilient cybersecurity frameworks using AI that protect it against current threats and also anticipate future challenges.

References

1. Z. Zhang, H. A. Hamadi, E. Damiani, C. Y. Yeun and F. Taher, "Explainable Artificial Intelligence Applications in Cyber Security: State-of-the-Art in Research," in IEEE Access, vol. 10, pp. 93104–93139, 2022, https://doi.org/10.1109/ACCESS.2022.3204051.
2. Strielkina, O. Illiashenko, M. Zhydenko and D. Uzun, "Cybersecurity of healthcare IoT-based systems: Regulation and case-oriented assessment," 2018 IEEE 9th International Conference

on Dependable Systems, Services and Technologies (DESSERT), Kyiv, UKraine, 2018, pp. 67–73, https://doi.org/10.1109/DESSERT.2018.8409101.
3. Radanliev, P., De Roure, D. Advancing the cybersecurity of the healthcare system with self-optimising and self-adaptative artificial intelligence (part 2). Health Technol. 12, 923–929 (2022). https://doi.org/10.1007/s12553-022-00691-6
4. de Azambuja, A.J.G.; Plesker, C.; Schützer, K.; Anderl, R.; Schleich, B.; Almeida, V.R. Artificial Intelligence-Based Cyber Security in the Context of Industry 4.0—A Survey. Electronics 2023, 12, 1920. https://doi.org/10.3390/electronics12081920
5. https://sloanreview.mit.edu/article/mayo-clinics-healthy-model-for-ai-success/
6. National Academy of Medicine; The Learning Health System Series; Grossmann C, Chua PS, Ahmed M, et al., editors. Sharing Health Data: The Why, the Will, and the Way Forward. Washington (DC): National Academies Press (US); 2022. 12, CASE STUDY: MAYO-GOOGLE PARTNERSHIP. Available from: https://www.ncbi.nlm.nih.gov/books/NBK594445/
7. https://www.healthcaredive.com/news/cleveland-clinic-creating-center-for-ai-in-healthcare/550370/
8. https://consultqd.clevelandclinic.org/how-ai-assists-with-staffing-scheduling-and-once-tedious-tasks

Chapter 5
AI and Healthcare Analytics

Contents

Abstract The incorporation of artificial intelligence (AI) and analytics in healthcare security is reforming the way healthcare organizations protect sensitive medical data. This paper explores the several uses of artificial intelligence and analytics in the field of healthcare security, as well as the revolutionary possibilities of machine learning and predictive analytics. By using these innovative tools, such as AI, medical practitioners may rapidly lower risk, proactively find weaknesses, and reinforce their cybersecurity system. One important topic addressed in this chapter is the application of machine learning to anomaly detection and security breach prediction. This will allow your system to be more resistant to possible attacks. The paper also provides several case studies of well-known healthcare firms that have effectively enhanced their safety through the use of artificial intelligence-powered analytics. Through a review of these instructive case studies, one may gain a deeper understanding of the development of cybersecurity in the medical industry. Moreover, one might gain additional knowledge on the advantages and disadvantages of using artificial intelligence for hospital security. The thorough case studies underline the critical role artificial intelligence and analytics play in safeguarding patient data and preserving the integrity of healthcare systems in a society where computers and digital systems are becoming more common.

S. Gupta et al., *Artificial Intelligence-Enabled Security for Healthcare Systems*,
https://doi.org/10.1007/978-3-031-82810-2_5

Keywords Healthcare security · Artificial intelligence · Patient data security · Advanced technologies in healthcare · Cybersecurity frameworks in healthcare · Regulatory compliance

5.1 Introduction

Within the healthcare field, technological advances in digital technology have greatly improved efficiency in patient care as well as in corporate procedures. Still, this has caused major privacy concerns as hackers have effectively accessed private patient information and big healthcare systems. Healthcare firms are improving their security systems through advanced data and artificial intelligence (AI) technology to handle these issues and improve usability. Including analytics and artificial intelligence in healthcare security has greatly improved cyberthreat detection, prevention, and eradication capabilities. These new techniques provide a chance to learn from the past and surpass the efficiency of their antiquated equivalents (Fig. 5.1).

At first, artificial intelligence (AI) was mostly used in medical research for data mining and pattern detection, therefore supporting healthcare security [2]. The field had a notable rise in the early 2000s, and the ability to do complex analysis of large-scale data increased. Security flaws have been more easily identified, indicating likely changes to machine learning systems during the next 10 years [3].

AI analytics became quite an important tool in the realm of defence in 2017. When medical professionals apply them, they may quickly see any weaknesses and start taking action to stop attacks.

Computer systems applying machine learning and other artificial intelligence techniques may examine enormous amounts of data and find trends suggesting the existence of security flaws. Using past data, these proactive security systems predict and block any hazards ahead.

AI analytics uses these methods to find data and system weaknesses, therefore allowing healthcare staff to apply preventative actions [5]. Several of the terms below show how analytics and artificial intelligence may improve healthcare safety.

Furthermore, discussed is the question of improved security measures these technologies offer for healthcare data systems. The exact uses of AI analytics and machine learning—more especially, their ability to improve threat detection and response capacity—are explored in this work. The benefits and drawbacks of using artificial intelligence-based security solutions in real-world situations are thoroughly reviewed in this paper. To do this, case studies of top-notch hospitals with successful application of such ideas are investigated. This paper also aims to show, by analysing both theoretical ideas and real-world examples, the relevance of artificial intelligence and analytics in guaranteeing the security of healthcare companies. Healthcare companies will be able to improve patient information security, follow laws, and keep the confidence of consumers and business partners in the digital sphere, where everything is interconnected in a digital atmosphere [6, 7].

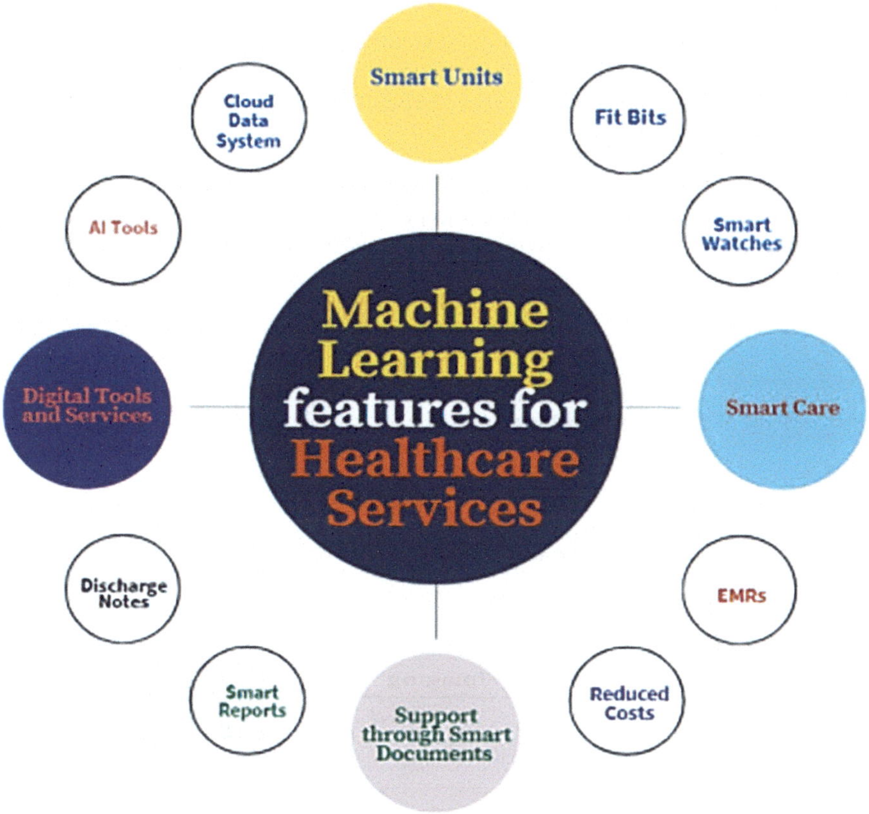

Fig. 5.1 Smart features of machine learning in the healthcare field [1]

5.2 Overview of the Use of AI and Analytics in Healthcare Security

Protecting patient data and guaranteeing faultless system operations depend on using artificial intelligence (AI) and analytics in healthcare security.

5.2.1 Necessity of AI and Analytics in Healthcare Security

The increasing frequency of attacks and the urgent need to protect private patient data make the use of artificial intelligence (AI) and analytics in healthcare security very necessary. The subsequent crucial factors that amplify the significance of this are given below.

Handling Large Volumes of Data
Compared to any other security solution, computer systems using artificial intelligence can quickly and efficiently examine more data. Using this method will help us to quickly spot complex and advanced cyberthreats [7] (Fig. 5.2).

Enhanced Threat Detection
By spotting to potential security breaches, machine learning algorithms help healthcare firms quickly and effectively react to possible security breaches. Usually, following this smart approach will help to minimize the damage caused by hackers [5, 7].

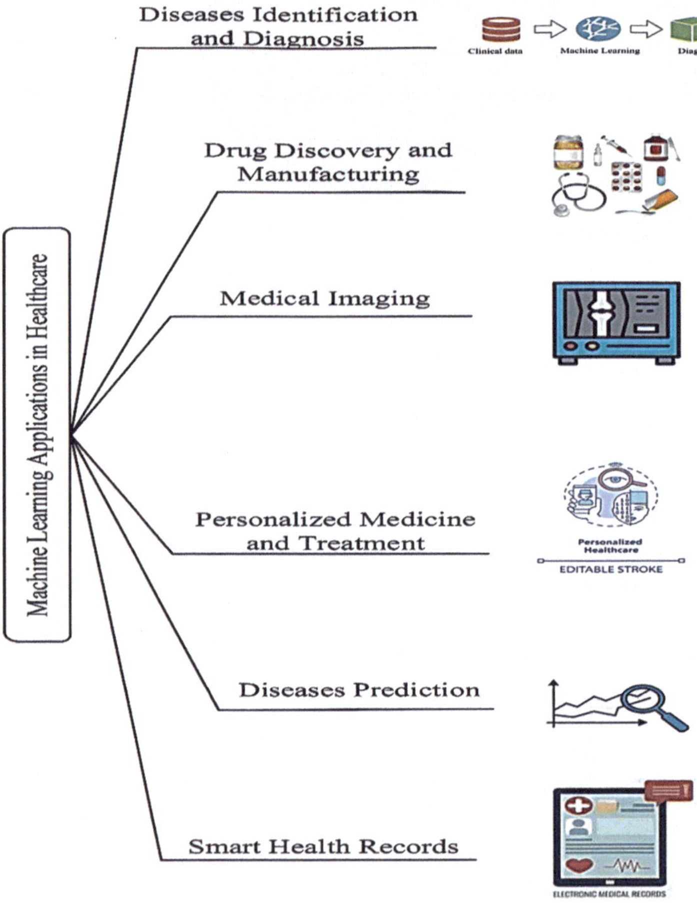

Fig. 5.2 Several AI/ML applications in the healthcare system [8]

5.2.2 *Predictive Analytics for Pre-emptive Security and Real-World Application*

Predictive analytics looks at past data to predict possible future threats and sites of security flaws. Consequently, healthcare facilities like hospitals can apply proactive strategies to improve general security and lower the possibility of data leaks [4, 5].

Automation of Security Processes
Artificial intelligence and analytics can help to effectively handle several security chores, including monitoring possible hazards, assessing vulnerabilities, and handling crises. This technology guarantees stability, accuracy, and speed, improving doctors' efficiency and stressing patient care [2].

Regulatory Compliance
Healthcare companies have to follow very important rules, like the Health Insurance Portability and Accountability Act (HIPAA). By constantly monitoring data access and usage, spotting illegal activities, and preserving thorough audit records, artificial intelligence (AI) and analytics help companies maintain compliance [4, 6].

Comprehensive Security Strategy
Natural language processing (NLP) is one area of artificial intelligence where unstructured data from different sources is examined to find possible vulnerabilities. Artificial intelligence (AI) technologies—including natural language processing (NLP)—helps to simplify data collection and interpretation from many sources. This raises the protection system's efficiency, therefore expanding its capability. These days, the complexity and range of cyber threats [3, 6] have grown, so an entire solution is needed.

5.2.3 *Anomaly Detection*

Adhering to regulations and employing artificial intelligence (AI) and analytics are essential for effectively mitigating the escalating complexity of cybersecurity threats in the healthcare sector. To ensure the confidentiality of sensitive patient data, it is essential to adhere to these steps. These technologies improve the stability and safety of the hospital environment by virtue of their ability to identify potential hazards, expedite security procedures, and implement proactive measures [6]. In this study, the main aspects of analytics and artificial intelligence (AI) in healthcare security are carefully looked into as they relate to previous research in the field (Table 5.1).

Table 5.1 Key Aspects of AI and Analytics in Healthcare Security

Aspect	Description
Enhanced threat detection	AI systems can analyse vast amounts of data in real-time to detect anomalies and potential threats that traditional methods might miss [7].
Predictive analytics	Leveraging historical data to forecast potential security breaches, enabling proactive measures [5].
Anomaly detection	Identifying deviations from normal behaviour that may indicate security incidents [3].
Automation of security processes	Automating threat monitoring, incident response, and risk assessment to improve efficiency and accuracy [2].
Role of natural language processing (NLP)	Analyzing unstructured data from security logs and incident reports to identify potential issues [6].
Enhanced data privacy and compliance	Ensuring compliance with regulations like HIPAA by monitoring data access and usage [4].
Incident response and recovery	Facilitating faster and more effective incident response and post-incident analysis [7].
Real-world applications	Case studies of healthcare organizations successfully implementing AI-driven security solutions [5].
Challenges and future directions	Addressing challenges such as investment, integration, and ethical concerns, and looking towards future advancements [3].

5.3 Challenges and Trade-Offs Between Privacy and Utility

Integrating analytics and AI into healthcare security presents some challenges, despite its advantages. These challenges encompass a significant upfront investment, the need to navigate integration with current systems, and addressing the societal implications that arise from AI implementation. However, privacy remains a paramount concern (Fig. 5.3).

Privacy-preserving machine learning (PPML) techniques are application-specific and cannot be generalized to all methods. As ML is an emerging field, new algorithms are introduced daily, requiring developers to develop novel methods for preserving privacy. Distributed approaches or local differential privacy (LDP) are often used, such as Microsoft's LDP for Windows 10 app tracking. However, most privacy-protection techniques cannot be directly adapted to new algorithms due to their specific use cases [10].

Scalability is another challenge, as high-processing-power algorithms can take more time and power for large datasets. ML is advancing towards low processing power, high communication costs, and better speed, but excessive computational power and communication costs are significant limitations. Distributed/parallel processing usage and transferring only the most important information to the algorithm can help [11].

Legibility is another challenge, as data owners should be informed about their data collection and privacy protection. Companies like Facebook, Google, and

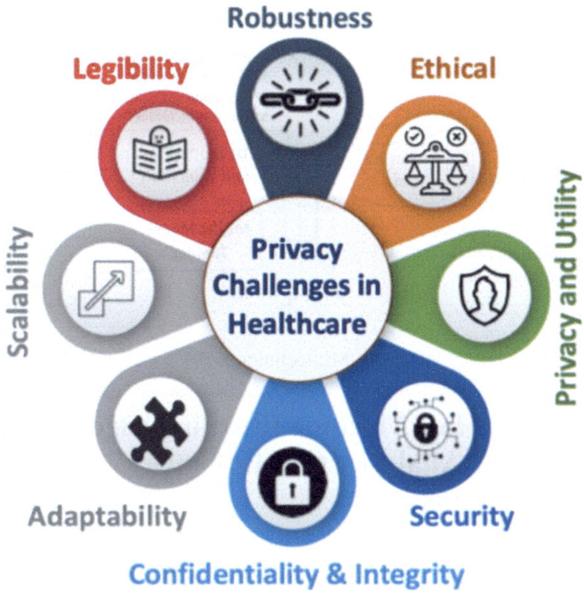

Fig. 5.3 Challenges towards building privacy-preserving AI in healthcare [9].

Amazon employ differential privacy for personal data storage, but it remains challenging to ensure users' data privacy is preserved [12].

AI ethics are crucial, as algorithms make crucial decisions affecting human lives. Ensuring fair, unbiased, and transparent algorithms is essential, as is protecting data integrity from data poisoning attacks. Robustness is also crucial, as models use data for crucial care decisions [13].

5.3.1 Trade-Off Between Privacy and Utility

Let's say a healthcare system wants to share its data but needs to remove the personal information from it first. They want to share information that is as correct as possible (minimize utility loss) and without bias (minimize justice loss). We can see that the trends of both justice and utility loss can change when we look at the results of both fake and real-world data in small chunks. This difference could be caused by a number of different data features. Because of this, it is very important to come up with ways to deal with the trade-off between privacy and usefulness. In the long run, it will help make things fairer and more private [9] (Fig. 5.4).

Future advancements in AI, such as improved machine learning models and more robust predictive analytics, hold promise for even more effective healthcare security solutions [3].

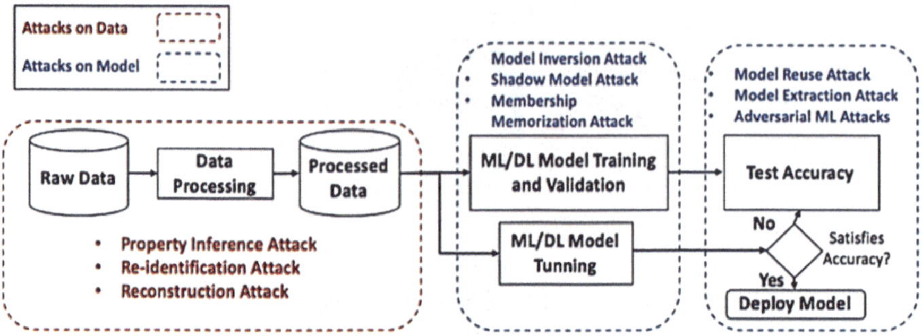

Fig. 5.4 Pipeline of the privacy attacks in ML techniques [9]

5.4 Discussion of How Machine Learning Algorithms and Predictive Analytics Can Enhance Healthcare Security

Predictive analytics and machine learning methods offer creative solutions to safeguard private patient data and healthcare systems, therefore increasing healthcare security. From better threat detection to proactive security measures, these technologies provide various benefits that significantly increase the defensive systems of healthcare organizations (Fig. 5.5).

5.4.1 Enhanced Threat Detection and Response

Machine learning techniques are essential for finding and reducing online threats in real time. These systems can look at huge amounts of data and find patterns and outliers that point to possible security holes (Fig. 5.6).

Some methods, like anomaly detection, can bring strange behavior to light so that it can be looked into further by telling the difference between normal and suspicious activities. Machine learning's ability to handle and analyse data at such a large and fast scale makes it much easier to find sophisticated cyber threats that might not be seen with traditional security methods [3, 15].

5.4.2 Predictive Analytics for Proactive Security

Predictive analytics forecasts future security occurrences using prior data, therefore helping healthcare industries act before the problem arises. By using trend detection and previous security event analysis, predictive models may project possible weaknesses and attack vectors. Defensive solutions used by healthcare providers enabled by predictive

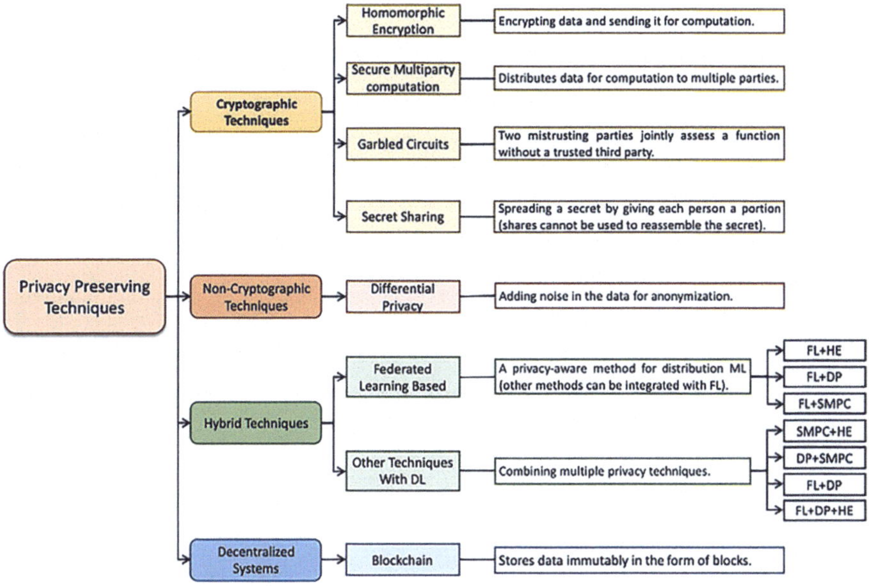

Fig. 5.5 Taxonomy of privacy-preserving techniques [14]. (Legends: *SMPC* Secure Multiparty Computation, *FL* Federated Learning, *DL* Deep Learning, *HE* Homomorphic Encryption, *DP* Differential Privacy)

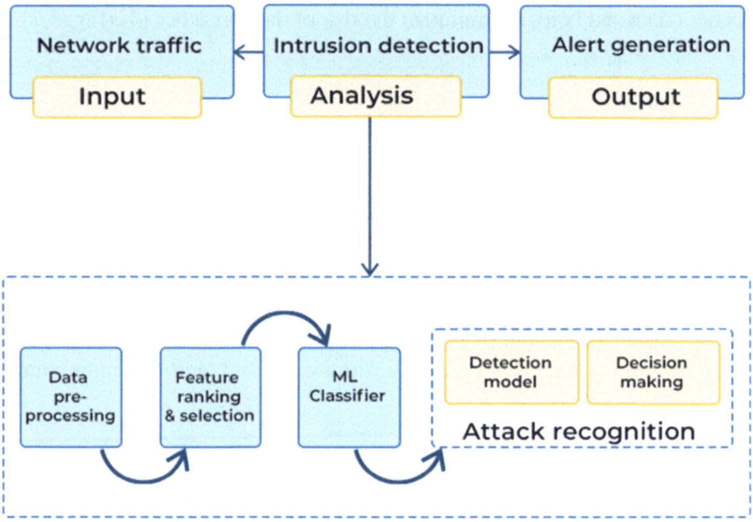

Fig. 5.6 System architecture of network anomaly detection system [14]

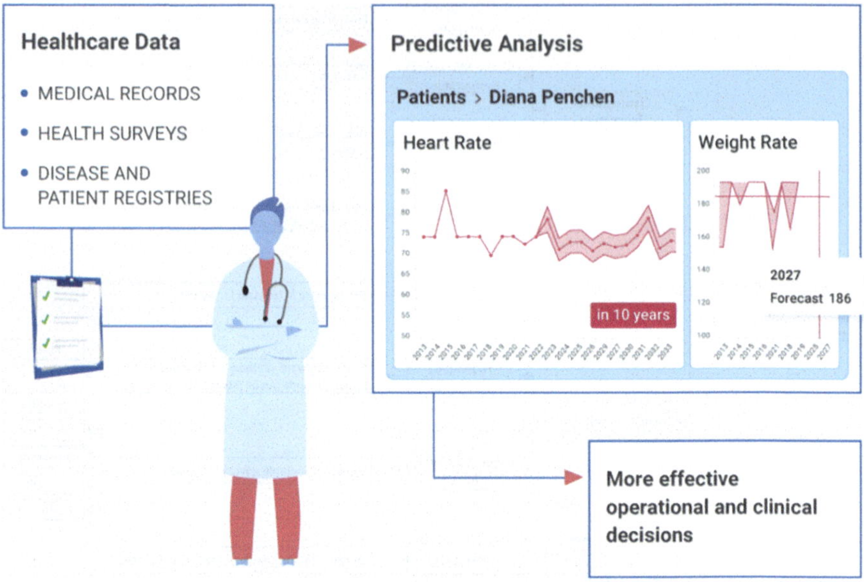

Fig. 5.7 Predictive analytics in healthcare [16]

analytics assist in establishing a proactive security posture by allowing them to implement them before a breach occurs. This proactive approach guarantees continual protection of patient data and helps to minimize the risk of data breaches [4] (Fig. 5.7).

5.4.3 Automation of Security Processes

Automation, powered by machine learning and predictive analytics, enhances the efficiency and accuracy of security operations. Automated solutions assist human security teams to be less busy by completing standard security tasks such as network traffic monitoring, risk analysis, and incident response. Automation not only improves operational efficiency but also provides consistency in security processes, which helps to maintain a robust security framework and facilitate maintenance [2].

5.4.4 Real-Time Threat Intelligence

Machine learning algorithms may interpret real-time data from multiple sources, therefore providing current risk information. This function allows health care organizations to change their security protocols and stay ahead of fresh hazards. Dynamic and adaptive security policies depend on real-time threat data, which enables the healthcare industry to react rapidly to new and evolving cyberthreats [6].

5.4.5 Enhanced Data Privacy and Compliance

Healthcare businesses have challenges complying with legislation and safeguarding data privacy. Machine learning and predictive analytics may assist by continuously monitoring data access and usage, detecting any illicit activities, and generating comprehensive audit logs. Subsequently, legislation such as the Health Insurance Portability and Accountability Act (HIPAA) relies on continuous surveillance. Nevertheless, ongoing research is being conducted to assess the potential of these technologies for facilitating regulatory compliance. This involves the automated detection and reporting of alleged privacy breaches, while ensuring the security of patient data [7].

5.5 Case Studies and Practical Applications

Several case studies have unequivocally demonstrated the advantages of using machine learning and predictive analytics into healthcare security. Hospitals have experienced a notable decrease in the duration required to detect and eradicate ransomware attacks by utilizing AI-driven methods for identification. AI-driven security framework successfully prevented a major data breach, illustrating the real-world impact of these technologies [5]. Machine learning methods and predictive analytics offer ground-breaking tools to enhance medical security. By way of improved threat detection, proactive security measures, mechanization of processes, and compliance assurance, these technologies provide a powerful defence against the widening terrain of cyber threats. As they maintain using and merging these innovative technologies, healthcare organizations might attain a superior degree of security, protecting patient information as well as the integrity of healthcare systems. Below are detailed case studies of organizations that have successfully implemented these technologies.

5.5.1 Case Study 1: Mayo Clinic's AI-Powered Cybersecurity Initiative

5.5.1.1 Organization: Mayo Clinic

Challenge: The Mayo Clinic, a leading nonprofit American academic medical centre, faced increasing cyber threats targeting its vast amounts of sensitive patient data. These attacks' frequency and complexity surpass those of the existing traditional security mechanisms.

Solution: Responding, the Mayo Clinic created a cybersecurity system with artificial intelligence drive. The AI-driven cybersecurity framework looked at network data using machine learning methods in search of unusual inclinations evocative of prospective attacks. Using predictive analytics based on historical data, they also anticipated potential future attacks.

Outcome: The time needed to identify and manage threats was thus substantially reduced. Real-time monitoring and anomaly identification made possible by the AI-powered system. Implementation of this AI system resulted in a 30% reduction in successful cyberattacks within the first year, demonstrating a substantial improvement in their cybersecurity posture [4].

5.5.2 *Case Study 2: Cleveland Clinic's Predictive Analytics for Proactive Security*

5.5.2.1 Organization: Cleveland Clinic

Challenge: The Cleveland Clinic, a renowned medical research centre and hospital, experienced challenges with maintaining data security amidst increasing cyber threats. The main problem with their current security methods was their reactive nature; often, they led to delayed reaction to attacks.

Solution: The Cleveland Clinic applied predictive analytics into their cybersecurity plan to make this possible. This includes using machine learning models to forecast future flaws and likely attack paths from past security data, so anticipating these problems, the clinic would move early to reinforce its defences.

Outcome: By using a more proactive security posture resulting from the predictive analytics methodology, the Cleveland Clinic was able to stop any assaults before they started. It was noted that the clinic clearly saw a decline in security events, with a 40% decrease in data breach attempts within 6 months of operation [4].

5.5.3 *Case Study 3: UPMC's Automated Incident Response System*

5.5.3.1 Organization: University of Pittsburgh Medical Centre (UPMC)

Challenge: UPMC, one of the largest healthcare providers in the United States, faced many challenges with the speed and efficiency of their incident response systems. The manual nature of these activities often resulted in delays in controlling security breaches, therefore increasing the possibility of data loss and system outages.

Solution: UPMC set up an artificial intelligence powered automatic incident response system to improve its cybersecurity posture. In this system, machine learning techniques allow for the automatic identification and reaction to security events. It monitored network activity constantly, found anomalies, and started pre-defined reaction systems without human involvement.

Outcome: The automated system greatly raised UPMC's security incident management capability. It was reported that the system's performance in managing events resulted in a 35% general impact of cyberattacks on their operations; the time needed to identify and react to threats was decreased by 50% [6].

These case studies highlight the transformative impact of AI and analytics on healthcare cybersecurity. By leveraging these advanced technologies, healthcare organizations can enhance their threat detection, response capabilities, and overall security posture, ensuring the protection of sensitive patient data and the integrity of their healthcare systems.

5.6 Conclusion

Artificial intelligence is revolutionizing healthcare in many aspects. From drug research to telemedicine that might drive their decisions, artificial intelligence is giving doctors real-time data and insights from medical tests. Although the application of artificial intelligence in healthcare causes certain issues, the advantages are very obvious. Artificial intelligence will become even more crucial in the future of healthcare as long as technology develops. Healthcare systems and safeguarding private patient data are now augmented by analytics and artificial intelligence applied jointly in healthcare security. by means of huge data analysis to find abnormalities and predict future vulnerabilities, therefore enabling proactive security measures and development of attack detection and response capability utilizing artificial intelligence and machine learning algorithms. Predictive analytics promotes preventative action and helps to improve this protection even more by foreseeing future hazards based on past data. Based on case studies, including those from the Mayo Clinic, Cleveland Clinic, and UPMC, cybersecurity posture, a lower incidence of breaches, and faster incident reaction times are increasing. These findings highlight the crucial role artificial intelligence and analytics play in building a strong and safe healthcare environment able to resist the complex and dynamic nature of cyber-nature and ensure security.

References

1. Javaid, Mohd, Abid Haleem, Ravi Pratap Singh, Rajiv Suman, and Shanay Rab. "Significance of machine learning in healthcare: Features, pillars and applications." *International Journal of Intelligent Networks* 3 (2022): 58–73.
2. Jiang, X., Chiu, D., & Tang, J. (2004). Data Mining Applications in Healthcare. Journal of Healthcare Informatics Research, 2(3), 57–68.
3. Obermeyer, Z., & Emanuel, E. J. (2016). Predicting the Future — Big Data, Machine Learning, and Clinical Medicine. New England Journal of Medicine, 375, 1216–1219.
4. Reddy, S., & Aggarwal, R. (2017). Predictive Analytics in Healthcare. Healthcare Management Review, 12(4), 78–85.

5. Rashid, A. (2020). The Role of AI in Healthcare Cybersecurity. Journal of Healthcare Informatics, 12(3), 45–58.
6. Chakraborty, S., Gupta, R., & Mitra, P. (2021). Machine Learning in Healthcare Security: An Overview. Healthcare Technology Letters, 8(1), 15–22.
7. Kaur, R., & Kaur, P. (2022). Predictive Analytics for Cybersecurity in Healthcare. International Journal of Healthcare Management, 15(2), 100–112.
8. Rahmani, Amir Masoud, Efat Yousef poor, Mohammad Sadegh Yousefpoor, Zahid Mehmood, Amir Haider, Mehdi Hosseinzadeh, and Rizwan Ali Naqvi. "Machine learning (ML) in medicine: Review, applications, and challenges." *Mathematics* 9, no. 22 (2021): 2970.
9. Khalid, Nazish, Adnan Qayyum, Muhammad Bilal, Ala Al-Fuqaha, and Junaid Qadir. "Privacy-preserving artificial intelligence in healthcare: Techniques and applications." Computers in Biology and Medicine 158 (2023): 106848.
10. Butpheng, Chanapha, Kuo-Hui Yeh, and Hu Xiong. "Security and privacy in IoT-cloud-based e-health systems—A comprehensive review." *Symmetry* 12, no. 7 (2020): 1191.
11. Al-Rubaie, Mohammad, and J. Morris Chang. "Privacy-preserving machine learning: Threats and solutions." *IEEE Security & Privacy* 17, no. 2 (2019): 49-58.
12. M. Al-Rubaie and J. M. Chang, "Privacy-Preserving Machine Learning: Threats and Solutions," in *IEEE Security & Privacy*, vol. 17, no. 2, pp. 49–58, March-April 2019, https://doi.org/10.1109/MSEC.2018.2888775.
13. Rasheed, Khansa, Adnan Qayyum, Mohammed Ghaly, Ala Al-Fuqaha, Adeel Razi, and Junaid Qadir. "Explainable, trustworthy, and ethical machine learning for healthcare: A survey." Computers in Biology and Medicine 149 (2022): 106043.
14. https://www.spiceworks.com/tech/networking/articles/network-behavior-anomaly-detection/ (retrive:5th July 2024, 19:15 PM)
15. Ahsan, Mustofa, Kendall E. Nygard, Rahul Gomes, Md Minhaz Chowdhury, Nafiz Rifat, and Jayden F. Connolly. "Cybersecurity threats and their mitigation approaches using Machine Learning—A Review." *Journal of Cybersecurity and Privacy* 2, no. 3 (2022): 527–555.
16. https://www.revealbi.io/blog/predictive-analytics-in-healthcare (retrieve 5th July 2024, 16:00 PM)

Chapter 6
Challenges and Risks of AI-Enabled Healthcare Security

Contents

Abstract Implementation of artificial intelligence (AI) into healthcare systems might totally change operational efficiency, diagnosis, and patient treatment. Still, this development has some challenges and possible risks, particularly in the sphere of healthcare security. Emphasizing important issues including regulatory adherence, data confidentiality, and ethical quandaries, this chapter explores the complex landscape of implementing AI-powered healthcare security solutions. The often-shifting regulations and standards make achieving regulatory compliance in healthcare data and AI applications a continual difficulty. Given the private nature of medical data and the rising danger of cyber-attacks, safeguarding data privacy is very vital. Furthermore, raising ethical questions raises probable biases in AI systems and the need for openness in decision-making driven by artificial intelligence. We propose to use a set of strategies, including strong regulatory conformance, advanced data encryption techniques, and the development of ethical guidelines for the application of artificial intelligence in healthcare, to solve these issues and lower the associated dangers. Addressing these issues early on would help to properly use AI in healthcare and guarantee patient confidence and security.

Keywords Artificial intelligence (AI) · Healthcare systems · Operational efficiency · Diagnosis · Patient treatment · Healthcare security · Regulatory adherence · Data confidentiality

S. Gupta et al., *Artificial Intelligence-Enabled Security for Healthcare Systems*,
https://doi.org/10.1007/978-3-031-82810-2_6

6.1 Introduction

Artificial intelligence (AI) in healthcare is bringing in a new era of medical innovation, enhancing the accuracy of diagnosis, customizing treatment regimens to particular patients, and simplifying operational operations. Predictive analytics, natural language processing, and machine learning, along with other AI technologies, are transforming healthcare delivery. Still, these developments raise some interesting issues and challenges, particularly in relation to healthcare security.

The following subjects will be discussed in this chapter: ethical issues, data protection, and legal compliance. It will also provide suggestions for handling and reducing these hazards. Using artificial intelligence in healthcare has resulted in quick developments and a rising appeal. Initial studies revealed that by allowing the examination of large datasets, artificial intelligence (AI) might improve clinicians' decision-making capacity [1] (Fig. 6.1).

Subsequent studies showing the application of artificial intelligence in disease detection have shown notable increases in both accuracy and speed [3]. However, the use of artificial intelligence in the healthcare industry also begs serious questions. Goodman and Miller were among the pioneers in 2017 in exploring the difficulties of using artificial intelligence in the healthcare industry. It underlined the need to change rules to fit technological developments [4] (Fig. 6.2).

In 2019, Price et al. mentioned and discussed the difficulties of guaranteeing compliance with changing rules in several countries [6]. Within the healthcare sector using artificial intelligence (AI), data security has become a major issue. Ksiazek first brought out in 2018 the heightened susceptibility in the healthcare industry to data leaks and cyberattacks [7]. McKinney et al. expanded this issue in 2020 by stressing the need for strong encryption and security policies to guard patient information from illegal access and cyberattacks [8].

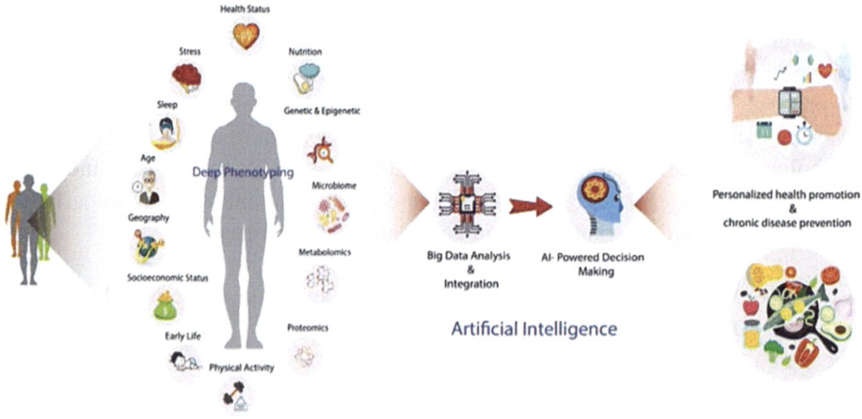

Fig. 6.1 Predictive analytics in healthcare [2]

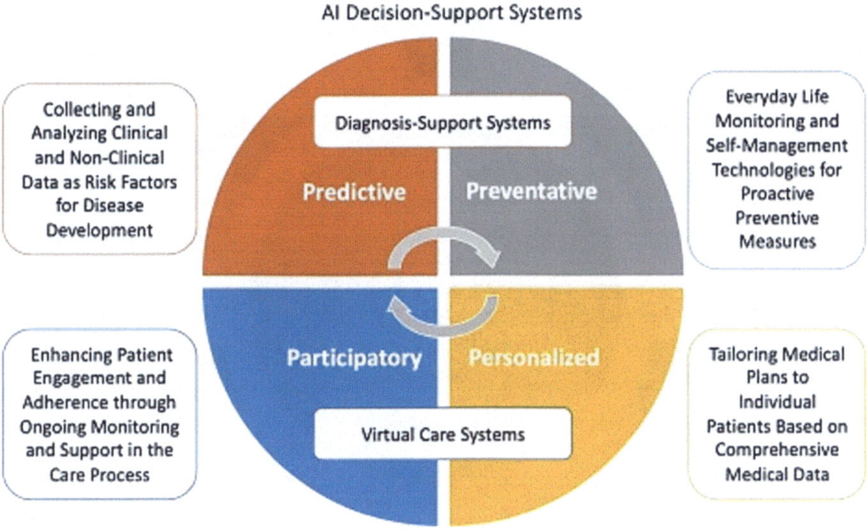

Fig. 6.2 Category and characteristics of AI decision-support systems [5]

The ethical consequences, like the possibility of prejudices in AI algorithms that might lead to unequal treatment and outcomes [9], should be one of top priority. The author underlined the need of developing moral values to ensure accountability and objectivity. More recently, the importance of transparency in artificial intelligence decision-making procedures has been underlined in order to support ethical standards and maintain patient confidence [10] (Fig. 6.3).

Many strategies have been proposed to help solve these problems. Regulatory alignment is the continuous effort of making sure AI systems are always changed to follow current laws and conventions. Protecting patient data depends mostly on strong security standards and reliable data encryption. Furthermore, putting strong ethical values into practice guarantees transparency in AI-powered healthcare and helps lower biases.

6.2 Potential Risk of Implementing of AI

Artificial intelligence (AI) integration into the healthcare industry raises various interesting challenges and possible risks, mostly related to adherence to regulatory requirements, protection of data privacy, and ethical considerations. To ensure the dependability and efficiency of artificial intelligence systems, these fields must be under exact control (Fig. 6.4).

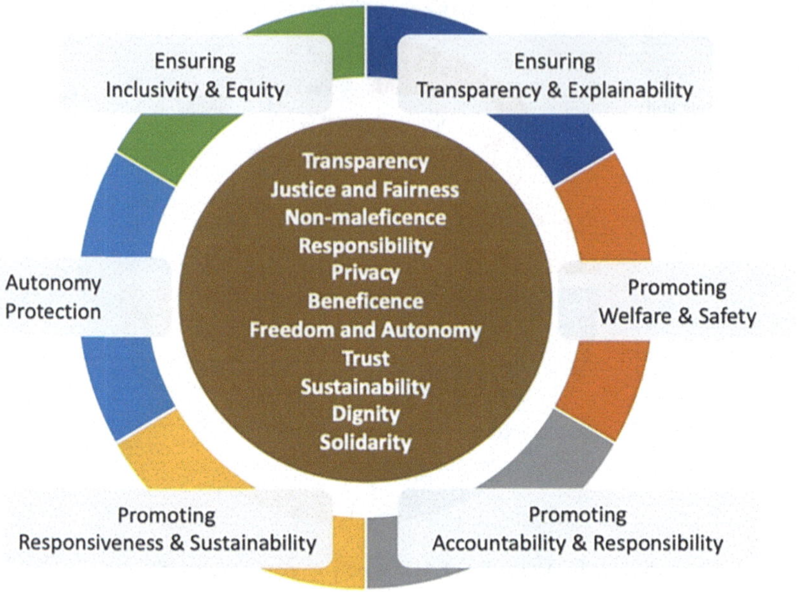

Fig. 6.3 Ethical principles and guidelines [5]

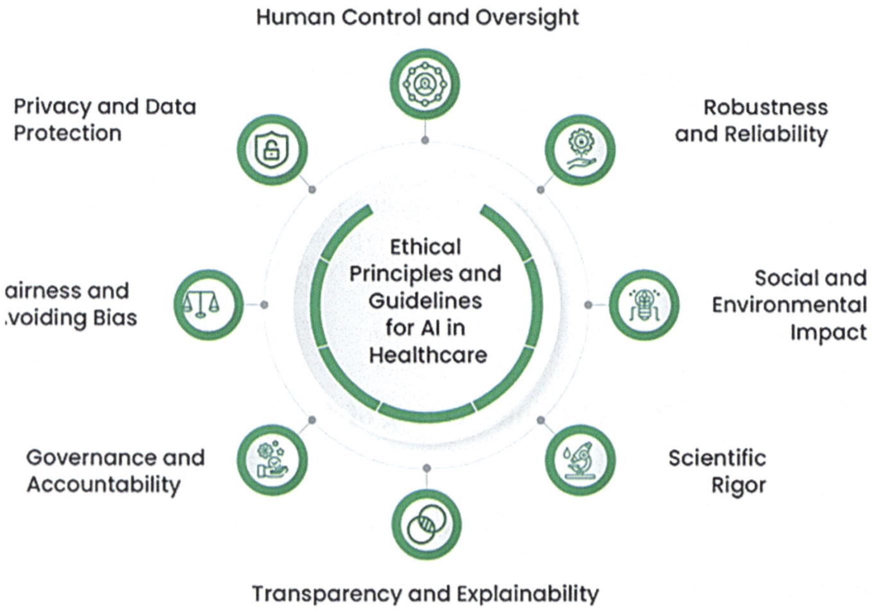

Fig. 6.4 Challenges of Implementing Responsible AI in Healthcare [11]

6.2.1 Regulatory Compliance

One of the main challenges in applying AI in healthcare is navigating the complex and growing regulatory landscape. To guarantee patient safety and data security, artificial intelligence systems in healthcare have to follow several rules. According to Goodman and Miller (2017), the current legal systems usually lack the required structure to properly handle the unique qualities of artificial intelligence technologies [4]. Thus, it is essential to change them and create new guidelines to solve issues unique to artificial intelligence.

6.2.2 Data Privacy

Data privacy is another serious concern when applying AI in healthcare. Effective operation of artificial intelligence systems usually depend on access to large amounts of personal health data. This material is of great secrecy; hence, its protection is absolutely vital.

Data collection and analysis helps AI systems unintentionally create privacy risks. One issue of concern is the prospect of re-identifying anonymized data sets, therefore compromising patient confidentiality. Using ever more advanced anonymizing and encryption methods is essential to reducing these risks. Still, it's important to always improve these strategies to successfully combat new dangers [8].

6.2.3 Ethical Considerations

Ethical considerations become the main focus when employing artificial intelligence in the healthcare system. The possibility that AI programs may be biased is one major issue. AI systems based on out-of-date data might unintentionally reinforce prejudices, leading to different treatment of different patient groups. As Challen et al. 2019 highlight, these biases can result from non-representative training data as well as from biased algorithmic design [9].

Regarding artificial intelligence decision-making processes, clarity is really crucial. Patients and doctors should clearly comprehend the decision-making process used by artificial intelligence systems if they are to build confidence and guarantee their correct use. The natural "black box" of many artificial intelligence systems might make it difficult to reach transparency. Establishing ethical guidelines and models will help to guarantee that artificial intelligence systems are built and used in a fair, open, and responsible way (Morley et al., 2020) [10].

6.3 Strategies for Addressing Challenges and Mitigating Risks

To address these challenges and mitigate the associated risks, several strategies can be employed:

- **Regulatory Alignment**: Maintaining current conformance to laws and standards depends on constant cooperation between artificial intelligence systems and regulatory authorities. In addition, to following the laws as they are, one should actively participate in developing new laws and rulese addressingg artificial intelligence technology.
- **Advanced Data Protection**: Modern encryption and anonymizing techniques help to protect patient information very well. To protect against always shifting cyber threats, regular security audits and updates are very necessary.
- **Ethical Frameworks**: Launching and adhering to strong ethical values guarantees transparency and helps to lower biases. This involves enhancing the transparency of algorithmic processes and training AI systems using diverse and inclusive data sets.
- **Ongoing Education and Training**: Artificial intelligence (AI) integration into healthcare systems presents various challenges largely related to data privacy protection, regulation adherence, and ethical issue resolution. To address these challenges, a thorough strategy including ethical frameworks, policy development, training, and technological solutions is required across all spheres.

- These techniques presented provide a whole approach for reducing security issues in AI-driven healthcare.

6.4 Roadmap for Mitigating the Risks Associated with AI-Enabled Healthcare Security

Artificial intelligence (AI) inclusion into healthcare systems presents various challenges, mostly related to data privacy protection, rule adherence, and ethical issue resolution. To address these challenges, a whole strategy, including ethical frameworks, policy development, and technical solutions, is required. The following solutions provide a comprehensive strategy for lowering security-related concerns in AI-powered healthcare.

6.4.1 Enhancing Regulatory Compliance

Healthcare companies have to have constant contact with regulatory agencies and be aware of developing rules to negotiate the complex regulatory terrain. Regarding this matter, a few points are discussed below.

- **Proactive Engagement**: Participating regularly in working groups and meetings with authorities helps one to exercise proactive engagement, therefore influencing the development of new rules and obtaining a better knowledge of them [6].
- **Compliance Frameworks**: Establishing strong internal compliance systems, including legal rules for the development and application of artificial intelligence technologies. These models should have enough adaptability to fit changes in regulations [4].

In 2018, the European Union (EU) passed a regulation under the General Data Protection Regulation (GDPR) to protect personal data under control by European Union-based data processors or controllers. It has set standards for notable legislative changes in Canada and the United States [12] (Fig. 6.5).

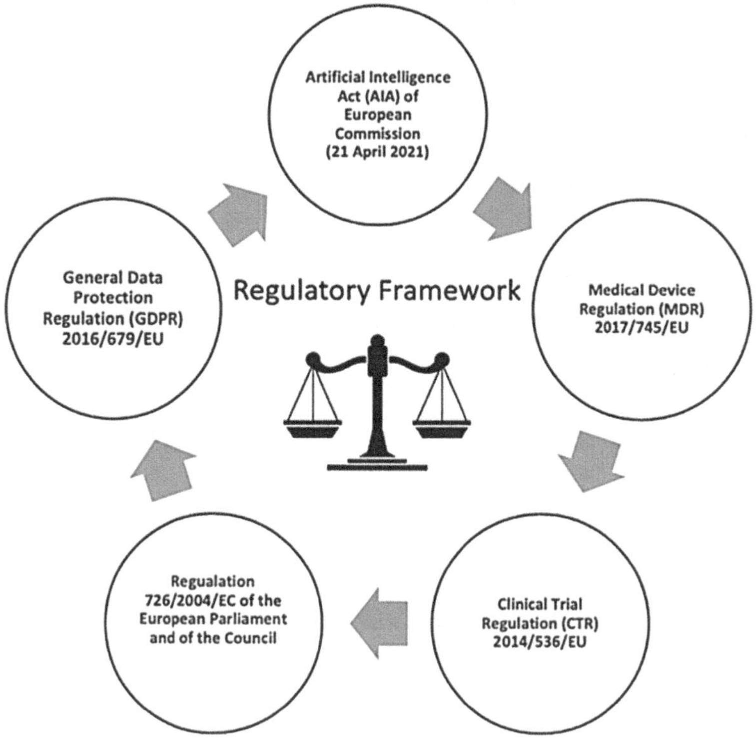

Fig. 6.5 Shows key European acts to govern AI in healthcare

Moreover, the European Commission has passed the Artificial Intelligence Act (AIA), meant to handle numerous issues resulting from the use of artificial intelligence [13, 14]. These rules aim to promote the deliberate use of artificial intelligence and minimize or stop any possible negative effects resulting from certain technological implementations. High-risk artificial intelligence systems are required under the proposed law to conduct pre-use compliance checks and post-market monitoring to guarantee adherence to the AIA policies [15].

The Food and Drug Administration (FDA) of the United States has started the process of creating rules controlling the application of artificial intelligence (AI) and machine learning in medical equipment. These rules underline the need to maintain reliability and openness in artificial intelligence systems. Yet, the rapid expansion of artificial intelligence often exceeds the ability of regulating authorities to adapt, which could result in gaps in monitoring [6].

In the United States, the Health Insurance Portability and Accountability Act (HIPAA) guarantees the protection and anonymity of medical data. Even with these rules in place, cyberattacks are getting more complex and consequently endanger data security more greatly [7].

6.4.2 *Strengthening Data Privacy Protections*

In the healthcare industry, data privacy is very important and calls for the protection of private patient data against illegal access and leaks. Good strategies include:

- **Advanced Encryption**: Advanced encryption is the application of the most recent encryption methods to guarantee data security either during storage or transmission. To properly combat developing threats [7], constant updating of encryption techniques is absolutely essential.
- **Anonymization and de-identification**: De-identification and anonymizing refer to applying strong methods to stop patient data from being rapidly reidentified. This lowers the possibility of privacy violations while allowing it to be used for artificial intelligence [8] training and analysis (Fig. 6.6).
- **Access Controls**: Access restrictions are the use of strong security and authentication systems to guarantee that only authorised people might view private data. Frequent audits and inspections help to efficiently find and stop illegal users of access.

6.4.3 *Developing Ethical Guidelines*

Adopting comprehensive regulations that guarantee rights, transparency, and responsibility in artificial intelligence (AI) systems can help overcome ethical problems. Among them, several important methods are:

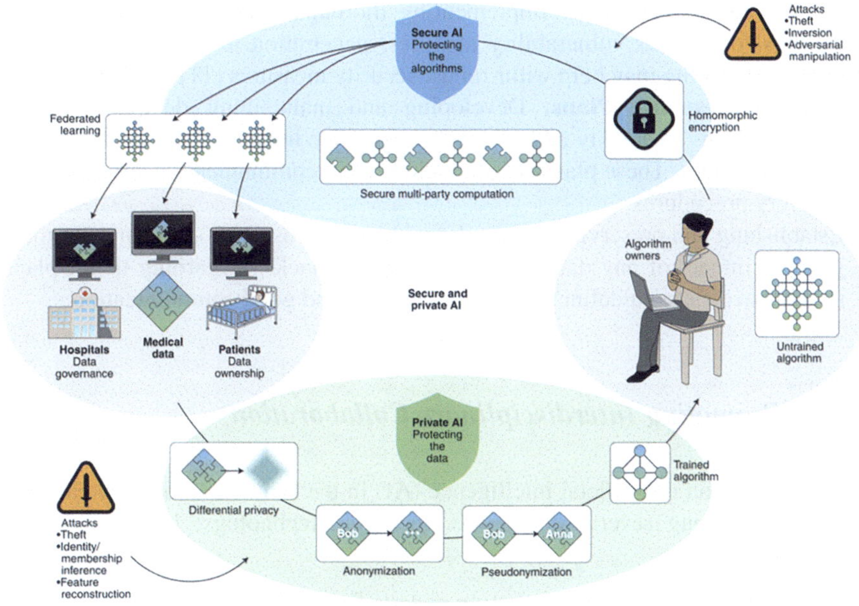

Fig. 6.6 Scematic overview of the relationships and interactions between data, algorithms, and techniques in the field of secure and private AI [11]

- **Bias Mitigation**: Using varied and broad datasets and guidance, AI systems help to proactively find and fix biases in them. Frequent testing of AI systems helps to find and fix any examples of bias [9].
- **Transparency and Explainability**: In artificial intelligence, maintaining transparency and explainability means making sure that AI systems' decision-making processes are transparent and understandable. This means creating artificial intelligence models that to give understandable justifications for their methods of decision-making. This builds patient and healthcare practitioner mutual confidence [10].
- **Ethical Training**: Providing ethical training for artificial intelligence developers, medical professionals, and other interested parties is advised. This helps to cultivate an attitude inside companies emphasizing accountability and transparency.

6.4.4 Implementing Robust Security Measures

Strong security mechanisms are required to protect artificial intelligence systems against cyberattacks and guarantee their best operation. Some are given below-

- **Cybersecurity Protocols**: Implementing thorough cybersecurity policy, and callings for regular vulnerability analyses, penetration testing, and real time threat monitoring may help withr robust security measures [11].
- **Incident Response Plans**: Developing and maintaining detailed incident response plans to quickly address and mitigate the impact of any data breaches or cyber-attacks. These plans should include clear communication strategies and recovery procedures.
- Establishing and preserving thorough incident response protocols can help mitigate the impact of any data breaches or cyber-attacks. Regarding these, plans should have clear guidelines for quick recovery and good communication.

6.4.5 Promoting Interdisciplinary Collaboration

Proper integration of artificial intelligence (AI) in the healthcare industry calls for cooperation among several disciplines, including technology, law, ethics, and medicine.

- **Interdisciplinary Teams**: Gathering experts from various fields into interdisciplinary teams to construct, operate, and supervise artificial intelligence systems. This cooperative strategy helps to solve the challenging issues related to artificial intelligence in the healthcare industry [4].
- **Stakeholder Engagement**: Incorporating several points of view and guaranteeing user happiness depend on the participation of several stakeholders, including patients, healthcare professionals, authorities, and developers of artificial intelligence [6].

- Through the implementation of these solutions, healthcare institutions might effectively solve the problems and reduce the dangers connected with AI-enabled healthcare security. This will guarantee ethical and safe application of these technologies as well as legal standards' compliance.

6.5 Conclusion

Artificial intelligence (AI) integration into the healthcare industry presents both great opportunities and significant challenges. AI raises important issues that must be properly addressed, even if it has the ability to revolutionize operational performance, diagnosis processes, and patient care. Ensuring conformity with rules is a big difficulty, as modern laws usually fall short of reflecting technological advancement. This calls for both ongoing updates and active participation with regulatory agencies. Because healthcare data is sensitive and cyber-attacks are becoming more likely, data privacy is a major issue. Strong anonymizing techniques, advanced encryption approaches, and rigorous access restrictions are very essential to guaranteeing patient data's security and confidence. Particularly in connection to probable biases in AI algorithms and the need of transparency in AI decision-making processes, the existence of ethical issues offers major challenges. Healthcare facilities have to adopt a multidisciplinary strategy, including the development and adherence to thorough ethical guidelines, assuring transparency in algorithms, and providing ongoing ethical training for all those engaged to lower these risks. These steps will help the healthcare industry effectively reduce the dangers related to artificial intelligence and maximize its revolutionary power. Although artificial intelligence-enabled healthcare has great promise, realizing its benefits calls for teamwork to overcome challenges and ensure the acceptable and moral application of AI technology in line with legal requirements.

References

1. Obermeyer, Z., & Emanuel, E. J. (2016). Predicting the future — big data, machine learning, and clinical medicine. *The New England Journal of Medicine*, 375(13), 1216–1219.
2. https://zenbit.tech/blog/ai-in-healthcare-advantages-and-disadvantages(Retrieve 7/7/2024, 20:01 PM)
3. Jiang, F., Jiang, Y., Zhi, H., Dong, Y., Li, H., Ma, S., ... & Wang, Y. (2017). Artificial intelligence in healthcare: past, present and future. *Stroke and Vascular Neurology*, 2(4), 230–243.
4. Goodman, K. W., & Miller, R. A. (2017). Ethics and regulatory challenges in the era of health information technology. *Journal of Law, Medicine & Ethics*, 45(2), 203–207.
5. Mennella, Ciro, Umberto Maniscalco, Giuseppe De Pietro, and Massimo Esposito. "Ethical and regulatory challenges of AI technologies in healthcare: A narrative review." Heliyon (2024).
6. Price, W. N., Gerke, S., & Cohen, I. G. (2019). Potential liability for physicians using artificial intelligence. *JAMA*, 322(18), 1765–1766.
7. Ksiazek, T. (2018). Protecting patient data: cybersecurity and data privacy in healthcare. *Journal of AHIMA*, 89(3), 44–47.
8. McKinney, S. M., Sieniek, M., Godbole, V., Godwin, J., Antropova, N., Ashrafian, H., ... & Reicher, J. J. (2020). International evaluation of an AI system for breast cancer screening. *Nature*, 577(7788), 89–94.
9. Challen, R., Denny, J., Pitt, M., Gompels, L., Edwards, T., & Tsaneva-Atanasova, K. (2019). Artificial intelligence, bias and clinical safety. *BMJ Quality & Safety*, 28(3), 231–237.
10. Morley, J., Floridi, L., Kinsey, L., & Elhalal, A. (2020). From what to how: an initial review of publicly available AI ethics tools, methods and research to translate principles into practices. *Science and Engineering Ethics*, 26(4), 2141–2168.
11. Kaissis, Georgios A., Marcus R. Makowski, Daniel Rückert, and Rickmer F. Braren. "Secure, privacy-preserving and federated machine learning in medical imaging." Nature Machine Intelligence 2, no. 6 (2020): 305–311.
12. Forcier M.B., Gallois H., Mullan S., Joly Y. Integrating artificial intelligence into health care through data access: can the gdpr act as a beacon for policymakers? *J. Law Biosci.* 2019;6:317–335. [PMC free article] [PubMed] [Google Scholar]
13. European Commission. European Commission; Brussels, Belgium: 2021. Proposal for a Regulation Laying down Harmonised Rules on Artificial Intelligence (Artificial Intelligence Act) p. 206. COM (2021) 206 final. [Google Scholar]

14. European Commission. 2021. Commission Staff Working Document, Impact Assessment, Accompanying the Proposal for a Regulation Laying down Harmonized Rules on Artificial Intelligence (Artificial Intelligence Act) p. 1. SWD (2021) 84 final, Part 1/2. [Google Scholar]
15. Schaake M. Standford Univeristy Human-Centered Artificial Intelligence (BHAI); Standford, Canada: 2021. The European Commission's Artificial Intelligence Act. 2021–06. [Google Scholar]

Chapter 7
Best Practices for Implementing AI-Enabled Healthcare Security

Contents

Abstract Artificial Intelligence if one end has empowered it to provide better healthcare, it has also created a widespread concern related to security and privacy like Phishing, Malware, Ransomware, Data Theft and Hacking of Iot Devices. This chapter aims to provide a complete view of various security concerns that arise in AI enabled healthcare systems by initially providing insights into explaining types of attack and mechanisms for cyber attacks with examples. Later in chapter Role of AI in healthcare security is explained in details by providing sufficient details about challenges and Risks in adoption of AI for healthcare. T he chapter further has necessary explanation about the best practices adopted in industry while adopting AI in healthcare whereby the concepts like backward integration, governance and Trust Frameworks.

Keywords Security · Governance · Healthcare · Cyberattacks · Trust frameworks · Artificial intelligence

S. Gupta et al., *Artificial Intelligence-Enabled Security for Healthcare Systems*,
https://doi.org/10.1007/978-3-031-82810-2_7

7.1 Introduction

Over the years, there has been a huge change in the healthcare system as it embraced Artificial Intelligence (AI). AI has transformed diagnosis and treatment of illness, administrative processes around healthcare and patient care. Artificial Intelligence (AI) has rapidly revolutionized the landscape of healthcare in wide areas such as patient care, diagnosis, treatment, and administrative processes [1]. The advancements come with significant concerns about security and privacy of patient information. The healthcare organizations collect enormous amount of data which is sensitive and prone for cyber-attacks [2]. The incredible breakthroughs come with quite grave worries on security and privacy. These medical institutions hold very sensitive details pertaining to patients hence their huge attraction for cyber-attacks. It is important that we understand the landscape of AI-enabled healthcare security to safeguard patient information and maintain the integrity of our health systems. Therefore, it is highly crucial to safeguard the data collected by various healthcare systems. The AI-enabled healthcare security systems provide crucial steps and solutions to safeguard patient information and maintain trust in the healthcare system. This chapter explores the best practices for designing and implementing AI-enabled healthcare security solutions, The solutions include integration of existing systems with establishing governance and trust frameworks that ensure data privacy and security [3, 4] (Fig. 7.1).

7.2 Healthcare Cyber Attacks

Healthcare cyber attacks pose significant threats to patient data security, the integrity of healthcare systems, and patient care delivery. These attacks can take various forms, targeting healthcare organizations' networks, medical devices, and electronic health records (EHRs). Here are some common types of healthcare cyber attacks (Fig. 7.2):

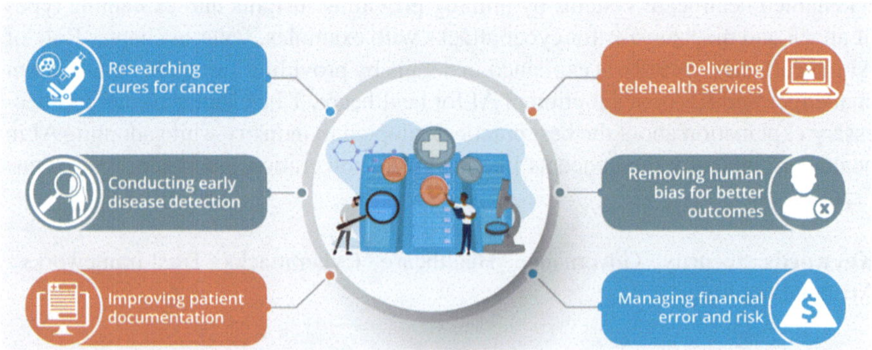
Researching cures for cancer
Conducting early disease detection
Improving patient documentation
Delivering telehealth services
Removing human bias for better outcomes
Managing financial error and risk

Fig. 7.1 Importance of healthcare data security [5]

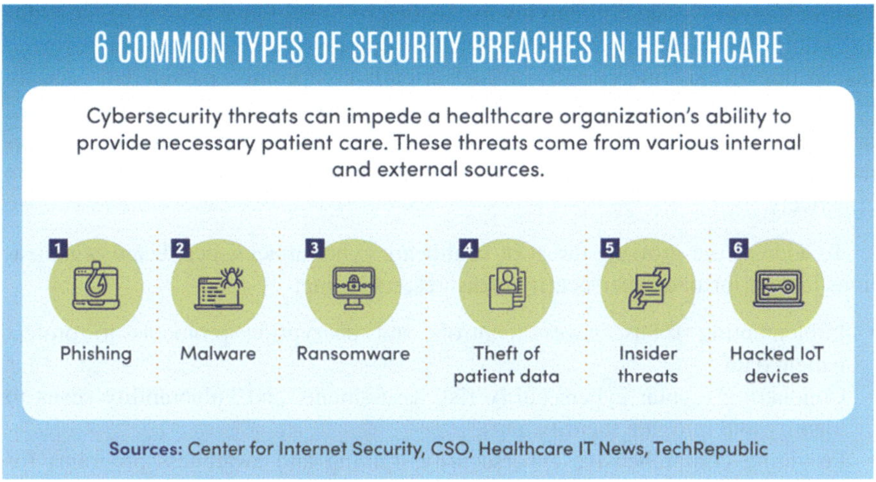

Fig. 7.2 Security breaches in healthcare

Ransomware Attacks Ransomware is a type of malware that encrypts data on a victim's system, rendering it inaccessible until a ransom is paid. Healthcare organizations are often targeted by ransomware attacks due to the sensitive nature of patient data and the critical role of healthcare services. Ransomware attacks can disrupt healthcare operations, compromise patient care delivery, and result in significant financial losses.

Data Breaches Data breaches involve unauthorized access to sensitive patient information, such as medical records, insurance details, and personal identifiers. Cybercriminals may exploit vulnerabilities in healthcare systems to steal patient data, which can be sold on the dark web or used for identity theft and fraud. Data breaches not only compromise patient privacy but also erode trust in healthcare organizations and expose them to regulatory penalties.

Phishing Attacks Phishing attacks involve the use of deceptive emails, messages, or websites to trick individuals into revealing sensitive information or downloading malicious software. Healthcare employees may be targeted with phishing emails posing as legitimate organizations or colleagues, leading to unauthorized access to healthcare systems and patient data. Phishing attacks can compromise the security of healthcare networks and facilitate further cyber threats.

Malware Infections Malware, including viruses, worms, and spyware, can infect healthcare systems and compromise their functionality. Malware infections can lead to system downtime, data loss, and unauthorized access to patient information. Cybercriminals may exploit vulnerabilities in outdated software or weak security controls to install malware on healthcare networks, posing significant risks to patient data security and healthcare operations.

Insider Threats Insider threats involve malicious or negligent actions by individuals within healthcare organizations, such as employees, contractors, or partners. Insider threats may intentionally or inadvertently compromise patient data security by accessing sensitive information without authorization, sharing login credentials, or falling victim to social engineering attacks. Healthcare organizations must implement robust access controls and monitoring mechanisms to mitigate insider threats effectively.

To address the growing threat of healthcare cyber attacks, healthcare organizations must prioritize cybersecurity measures, including:

- Implementing robust access controls and encryption protocols to protect patient data.
- Conducting regular cybersecurity risk assessments and vulnerability scans to identify and mitigate security gaps.
- Providing comprehensive cybersecurity training and awareness programs for employees to recognize and respond to cyber threats effectively.
- Establishing incident response plans and protocols to quickly detect, contain, and mitigate the impact of cyber attacks.
- Collaborating with cybersecurity experts, industry partners, and government agencies to share threat intelligence and best practices for enhancing healthcare cybersecurity.

By proactively addressing cybersecurity risks and implementing effective security measures, healthcare organizations can better safeguard patient data, maintain the integrity of healthcare systems, and ensure the delivery of safe and secure patient care (Fig. 7.3).

7.2.1 Magnitude and Financial Implication of Cyberattacks that Occurred Across the World

Cyberattacks are a growing threat, causing significant financial losses globally. The magnitude varies greatly, with some attacks crippling major infrastructure and costing billions, while others target individuals or smaller businesses. Regardless of size, cyberattacks disrupt operations, damage reputations, and result in hefty financial burdens for victims, highlighting the critical need for robust cybersecurity measures.

7.2.2 Examples of Healthcare Cyberattacks

The WannaCry Epidemic The 2017 WannaCry ransomware attack serves as a stark reminder of the potential consequences of inadequate cybersecurity measures in healthcare. This global incident disrupted operations in countless hospitals, high-

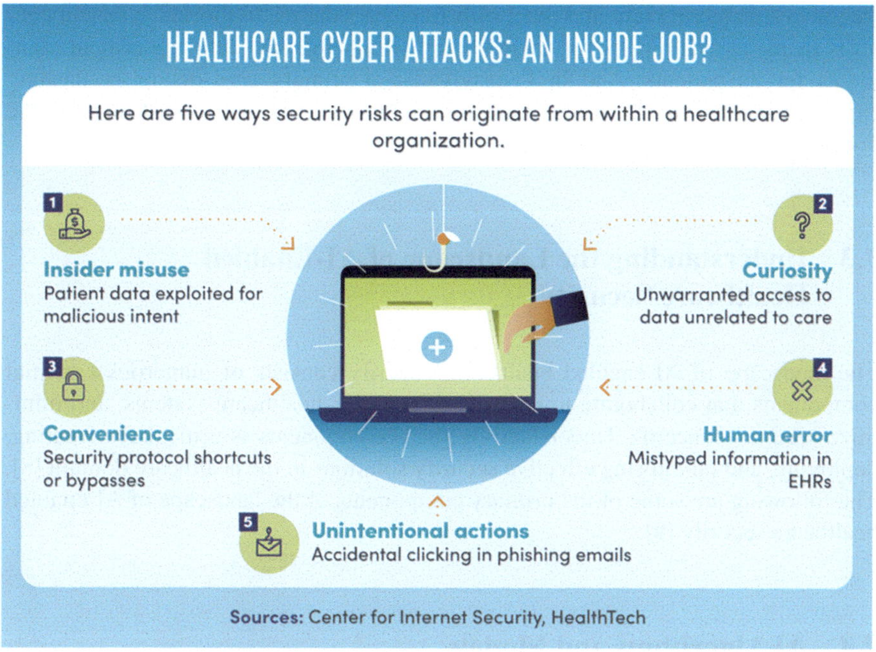

Fig. 7.3 Healthcare cyber attacks

lighting vulnerabilities in outdated software and lax cybersecurity practices. Patient records were compromised, appointments cancelled, and critical medical services temporarily halted. The incident underscored the urgent need for robust cybersecurity protocols to safeguard patient data and ensure the smooth functioning of healthcare facilities The impact of the WannaCry ransomware attack extended to the United Kingdom's National Health Service (NHS), resulting in significant disruption that led to the cancellation of more than 19,000 medical appointments. The estimated financial toll on the NHS was reported to be approximately £92 million ($120 million) [5].

India India recorded the second highest number of attacks, with a total of 7.7% of the total attacks on the healthcare industry in 2021. AIIMS hospital, the premier public hospital in India, was targeted by cyber attackers in November' 22. The attack forced the hospital to switch to Manual mode for 2 weeks. An estimated 1.3 Terabyte of data was encrypted. This affected 30–40 million patient data base which included prominent politicians of the country [6].

U.S. Health Care Payment System Cyberattack Paralyzes the Largest U.S. Health Care Payment System: The hacking shut down the nation's biggest health care payment system, causing financial chaos that affected a broad spectrum ranging from large hospitals to single-doctor practices. An urgent care chain in Ohio may be forced to stop paying rent and other bills to cover salaries. In Florida, a cancer center is racing to find money for chemotherapy drugs to avoid delaying critical treatments for its patients. And in Pennsylvania, a primary care doctor is slashing expenses and pooling all of her cash — including her personal bank stash — in the hopes of staying afloat for the next 2 months [7].

7.3 Understanding the Landscape of AI-Enabled Healthcare Security

The landscape of AI-enabled healthcare security consists of numerous essential components that collaborate to protect patient data, healthcare systems, and minimize security concerns. Understanding these components is critical for creating, deploying, and monitoring effective security solutions in the healthcare domain [8]. The following are some of the primary components of the landscape of AI-enabled healthcare security [9]:

7.4 AI Algorithms and Models

AI models and algorithms are the cornerstone of AI-enabled healthcare security systems. These algorithms cover a wide range of methods, including computer vision, natural language processing, deep learning, and machine learning. In healthcare security, machine learning techniques are frequently utilized for anomaly detection, pattern recognition, and predictive analytics. For image analysis and medical picture classification, deep learning models like convolutional neural networks (CNNs) and recurrent neural networks (RNNs) are used. Medical records, clinical notes, and research articles contain unstructured text data that is processed using natural language processing (NLP) techniques. Semantic analysis, entity recognition, and sentiment analysis are made possible by these algorithms to find information pertaining to security. Medical pictures, including X-rays, MRIs, and CT scans, are analyzed using computer vision algorithms to look for anomalies and disorders.

7.5 Data Sources and Inputs

The unprocessed data needed to train AI models and algorithms is provided by data sources. Digital health records (EHRs), lab test results, medical imaging data, patient demographics, and administrative data are some examples of data sources in the context of healthcare security. IoT sensors, wearable technology, health monitoring systems, and external databases that hold details on known security risks, vulnerabilities, and attack patterns are examples of additional data sources. Preparing the data for AI model training and feature extraction for security analysis involves applying data preparation techniques such data cleansing, normalization, and feature engineering.

7.6 Security Applications and Use Cases

A broad range of applications and use cases are covered by AI-enabled healthcare security solutions, which are designed to handle the different security threats and problems that healthcare organizations confront. Threat identification, detection of anomalies, fraud detection, intrusion detection, malware detection, risk assessment, control of access, authentication and authorization, and security monitoring are examples of common security applications. These apps use artificial intelligence (AI) models and algorithms to evaluate medical data, spot unusual activity, pinpoint security flaws, and offer practical advice for reducing security risks.

7.7 Integration with Healthcare Systems

Effective deployment of AI-enabled security solutions within healthcare organizations requires integration with current healthcare systems. Electronic health record (EHR) systems, pharmacy information systems, picture archiving and communication systems (PACS), hospital information systems (HIS), laboratory information systems (LIS), and medical device networks are a few examples of these systems. Interoperability, data interchange, and conformance with current standards, protocols, and infrastructure are all aspects of integration. To guarantee smooth integration and minimal interference with clinical procedures, cooperation with IT departments, system administrators, and healthcare experts is also necessary.

1. **Governance and Compliance:**
   - Governance and compliance frameworks play a crucial role in ensuring the ethical, legal, and regulatory compliance of AI-enabled healthcare security solutions.
   - Healthcare organizations must adhere to various regulations and standards, such as the Health Insurance Portability and Accountability Act (HIPAA), General Data Protection Regulation (GDPR), Health Information Technology for Economic and Clinical Health (HITECH) Act, and other industry-specific regulations.
   - Governance frameworks define policies, procedures, roles, responsibilities, and accountability mechanisms for managing security risks, protecting

patient privacy, and ensuring the responsible use of AI technologies in healthcare.

2. **Trust and Transparency:**

    - Trust and transparency are essential for fostering confidence in AI-enabled healthcare security solutions among healthcare providers, patients, regulators, and other stakeholders.
    - Trust frameworks establish principles, guidelines, and mechanisms for building trust in AI algorithms, models, and systems. These frameworks emphasize transparency, accountability, fairness, reliability, and explainability of AI-driven decision-making processes.
    - Transparency initiatives involve providing insights into the functioning of AI algorithms, disclosing data sources, methodologies, assumptions, limitations, and potential biases. This transparency enables stakeholders to understand how AI-enabled security solutions work, assess their performance, and make informed decisions about their deployment and use.

3. **Training and Education:**

    - Training and education programs are essential for building the knowledge, skills, and capabilities required to develop, deploy, and manage AI-enabled healthcare security solutions.
    - Healthcare professionals, IT staff, security professionals, data scientists, and other stakeholders need specialized training in AI technologies, cybersecurity principles, healthcare regulations, data privacy laws, and ethical considerations.
    - Training programs may include workshops, seminars, online courses, certifications, and hands-on exercises tailored to the specific needs and roles of different audiences within healthcare organizations.

4. **Continuous Monitoring and Improvement:**

    - Continuous monitoring and improvement are essential for maintaining the effectiveness, efficiency, and relevance of AI-enabled healthcare security solutions over time.
    - Monitoring involves real-time surveillance, analysis, and reporting of security events, incidents, and performance metrics. It enables proactive detection of security threats, timely response to security incidents, and ongoing optimization of security controls.
    - Improvement involves iterative refinement of AI algorithms, models, and systems based on feedback, data insights, lessons learned, and emerging trends in healthcare security. It also involves regular updates, patches, and enhancements to address new security threats, vulnerabilities, and regulatory requirements.

Thus, the landscape of AI-enabled healthcare security comprises various components, including AI algorithms and models, data sources and inputs, security applications and use cases, integration with healthcare systems, governance and compliance, trust and transparency, training and education, and continuous monitoring and improvement. These components work together to address security challenges, mitigate risks, and safeguard patient data in the rapidly evolving healthcare environment.

7.7.1 The Role of AI in Healthcare Security

Artificial intelligence (AI) has made important advances in a variety of fields, including healthcare. With the increasing digitization of medical records and the increased threat of cyber attacks, artificial intelligence has emerged as a viable tool for securing medical data and patient privacy.AI plays an integral part in healthcare cybersecurity by protecting medical data and patient privacy. Healthcare businesses can improve their entire cybersecurity posture and reduce the risks associated with cyber assaults by implementing AI systems for threat detection, anomaly detection, and access control.AI plays a pivotal role in enhancing healthcare security by providing advanced tools and techniques for threat detection, anomaly detection, and predictive analytics.AI systems can analyze large amounts of data swiftly and accurately, allowing healthcare businesses to recognize possible security issues and take proactive measures to minimize them. AI can help detect and prevent breaches before they happen by constantly monitoring network traffic and discovering trends that indicate a cyber attack is underway [9].

One of the most significant advantages of AI in cybersecurity is its capacity to adapt and learn from new threats. Traditional security methods sometimes rely on predefined rules and signatures, rendering them ineffective against acquiring and sophisticated threats. AI, on the other hand, can constantly learn from fresh data and upgrade its algorithms in order to recognize and react to emerging risks.

AI also excels at anomaly detection. By establishing a baseline of normal behavior, AI can immediately identify and highlight any odd or questionable action. This can help healthcare firms uncover insider risks or unlawful access to sensitive patient data. AI can improve the effectiveness of authorization and authentication systems. AI can examine user behavior and find anomalies that could signal a compromised account using machine learning techniques. This can help to prevent illegal access and keep patient data from falling into the wrong hands. While AI can provide considerable benefits in healthcare cybersecurity, it is critical to establish a balance between security and privacy. Ensuring that AI systems adhere to rules and ethical principles is critical to safeguarding patient confidentiality [10].

AI in healthcare cybersecurity is critical for securing clinical data and preserving confidentiality for patients. As technology has become more prevalent in the medical field, so has the possibility of cyber threats. AI provides various advantages that can help reduce these risks and protect the confidentiality of delicate healthcare data. AI in healthcare cybersecurity has various advantages that are critical for securing medical data and patient privacy. From improved threat detection and prevention to proactive risk management and quick response to incidents, AI technology is critical to guaranteeing healthcare system security and integrity. Healthcare firms may boost their cybersecurity defenses and keep the trust of patients as well as partners by harnessing AI's capabilities [11].

AI Healthcare Benefits

- **Enhanced Threat Detection and Prevention:** One of the most important advantages of AI in healthcare cybersecurity is its capacity to detect and block threats more efficiently. Systems fueled by AI are able to evaluate massive volumes of data in real time, allowing them to detect potential security flaws and malicious activity quickly. AI can detect anomalies and inform security professionals to take fast action, averting potential data breaches.
- **Proactive Risk Management:** AI technology can proactively detect flaws in health care facilities and networks, allowing firms to repair them before they are exploited by hackers. AI can assess the privacy posture of the medical system using sophisticated mathematical models and machine learning, identifying flaws and recommending fixes. This proactive approach allows healthcare firms to stay one step beyond emerging risks and reduces the chance of data breaches.
- **Efficient incident handling:** In the event of a security problem, AI can dramatically improve the incident response procedure. AI-powered systems can detect and respond to security breaches automatically, allowing for a quick and effective response time. By evaluating past data and patterns, AI may deliver significant insights into the type and severity of an event, allowing security professionals to take proper action to limit and mitigate the intrusion.
- **Continuous surveillance and Dynamic Security**: AI provides continuous monitoring of healthcare systems and networks, ensuring 24/7 defense against cyber attacks. Machine learning allows AI systems to adapt and evolve in response to new threats and trends in attacks, resulting in them being more successful in protecting medical information and patient privacy. This dynamic security solution ensures that healthcare organizations remain safe from new hazards in an ever-changing cybersecurity landscape.

7.7.2 Challenges and Risks

Despite the numerous benefits of AI-enabled healthcare security, there are also several challenges and risks that need to be addressed. One of the primary challenges is the sheer volume and complexity of healthcare data. Healthcare organizations generate massive amounts of data from various sources, including electronic health records (EHRs), medical imaging, wearable devices, and IoT sensors. Managing and securing this data presents significant challenges, particularly in ensuring its integrity, confidentiality, and availability.

Another challenge is the lack of skilled cybersecurity professionals with expertise in AI technologies. The field of AI-enabled healthcare security is relatively new and rapidly evolving, making it difficult for organizations to find qualified professionals who can effectively design, implement, and manage AI-powered security solutions. Moreover, there is a shortage of standardized training programs and educational resources for healthcare professionals interested in pursuing careers in cybersecurity.

Furthermore, the interconnected nature of healthcare systems and the proliferation of connected devices increase the attack surface for cybercriminals. Healthcare organizations must contend with a wide range of security threats, including ransomware attacks, data breaches, insider threats, and malware infections. Moreover, the interconnectedness of healthcare systems poses challenges in terms of interoperability, data sharing, and maintaining the privacy and security of patient information across disparate systems [12] (Fig. 7.4).

7.8 Best Practices for Designing and Implementing an AI-Enabled Healthcare Security Solution

Designing and implementing an AI-enabled healthcare security solution requires a comprehensive approach that addresses various aspects, including integration with existing systems, establishment of governance and trust frameworks, and ensuring data privacy and security. By following these best practices for designing and implementing an AI-enabled healthcare security solution, healthcare organizations can effectively integrate with existing systems, establish governance and trust frameworks, and ensure data privacy and security in the rapidly evolving healthcare landscape. These practices help mitigate security risks, protect patient information, and maintain the integrity and confidentiality of healthcare systems and data (Fig. 7.5).

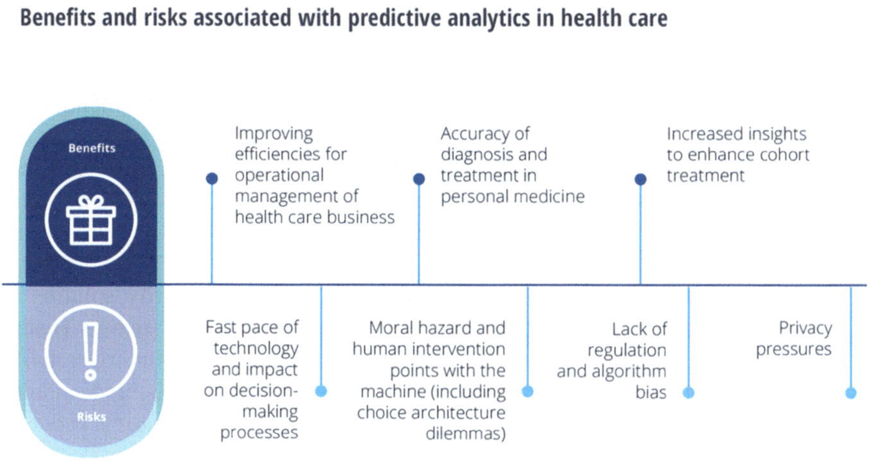

Fig. 7.4 Benefits and risk of predictive analysis in healthcare

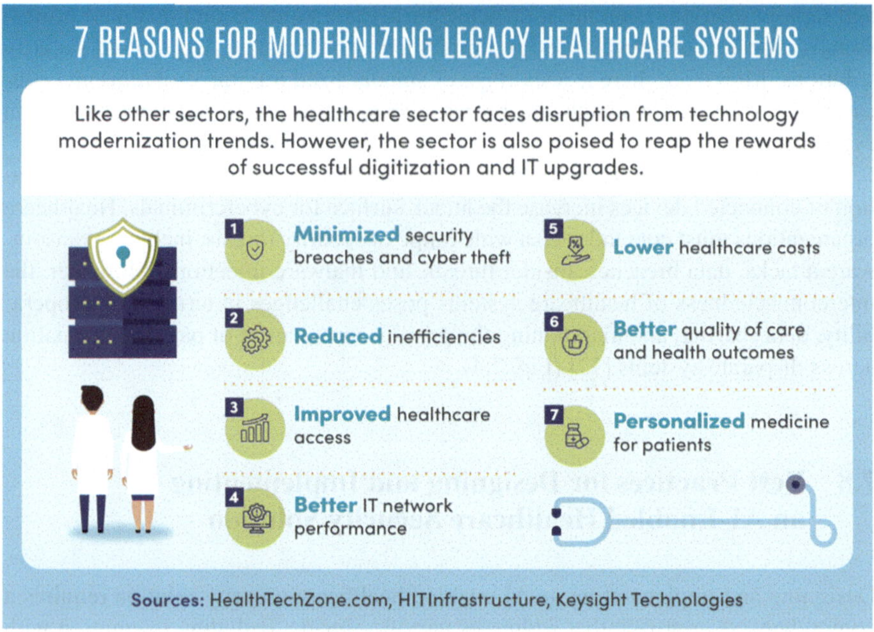

Fig. 7.5 Modernizing healthcare systems

Below are best practices for each of these components [13]:

1. **Integration with Existing Healthcare Systems:** With the growing use of artificial intelligence (AI) in healthcare, preserving medical data and patient privacy have become crucial considerations. Implementing the aforementioned suggestions would allow healthcare businesses to effectively integrate AI into their cybersecurity processes, assuring the confidentiality of clinical data and patient privacy. As AI advances, prioritizing cybersecurity is critical to maintaining trust and confidence in healthcare systems.

   - **Conduct a Comprehensive System Assessment:** Before implementing an AI-enabled security solution, conduct a thorough assessment of existing healthcare systems, including electronic health records (EHRs), hospital information systems (HIS), and other IT infrastructure. Identify integration points, data flows, interoperaility requirements, and potential compatibility issues.
   - **Ensure Interoperability:** Ensure that the AI-enabled security solution is compatible with existing healthcare systems and standards, such as Health Level Seven International (HL7) and Fast Healthcare Interoperability Resources (FHIR). Implement data exchange protocols, APIs, and middleware solutions to facilitate seamless integration and data sharing between different systems.

- **Customize Integration Solutions:** Tailor integration solutions to meet the specific needs and requirements of healthcare organizations. Consider factors such as data formats, data mapping, data transformation, message routing, and error handling to ensure smooth operation and minimal disruption to clinical workflows.
- **Collaborate with IT Departments:** Collaborate closely with IT departments, system administrators, and other stakeholders to plan and execute integration activities effectively. Involve IT personnel in the design, development, testing, and deployment phases to address technical challenges and ensure the successful implementation of the AI-enabled security solution.
- **User Training and Awareness**: Inform healthcare professionals and employees about cybersecurity best practices. Education initiatives can assist them comprehend the necessity of securing patient data while also teaching them how to recognize and prevent possible safety risks.
- **Collaboration and Information Sharing:** Encourage collaboration among healthcare organizations and cybersecurity professionals. Sharing knowledge and recommendations will help organizations keep current on the newest cybersecurity dangers and protective measures.
- **Regulatory Compliance**: Comply with legal and regulatory regulations governing healthcare data privacy and security. Compliance with regulations like HIPAA guarantees that information regarding patients is handled safely and confidentiality is protected.

2. **Establishment of Governance and Trust Frameworks** [14]:

- **Define Clear Governance Structures:** Establish clear governance structures, policies, and procedures to oversee the design, implementation, and management of the AI-enabled security solution. Define roles, responsibilities, decision-making processes, and accountability mechanisms to ensure effective governance and compliance with regulatory requirements.
- **Develop Trust Frameworks:** Develop trust frameworks to build confidence in the AI-enabled security solution among stakeholders, including healthcare providers, patients, regulators, and other parties. Emphasize transparency, accountability, fairness, reliability, and explainability in AI-driven decision-making processes. Provide visibility into the functioning of AI algorithms, data sources, methodologies, assumptions, limitations, and potential biases to enhance trust and transparency.
- **Establish Risk Management Processes:** Implement risk management processes to identify, assess, mitigate, and monitor security risks associated with the AI-enabled security solution. Conduct regular risk assessments, vulnerability scans, penetration tests, and security audits to identify potential threats, vulnerabilities, and weaknesses. Develop risk mitigation strategies, contingency plans, and incident response procedures to address security incidents and minimize their impact on healthcare operations.
- **Ensure Compliance with Regulations:** Ensure compliance with relevant regulations, standards, and guidelines governing healthcare security, data pri-

vacy, and AI technologies. Familiarize yourself with regulations such as the Health Insurance Portability and Accountability Act (HIPAA), General Data Protection Regulation (GDPR), Health Information Technology for Economic and Clinical Health (HITECH) Act, and other industry-specific requirements. Implement controls, safeguards, and measures to protect patient data, ensure confidentiality, integrity, and availability, and prevent unauthorized access or disclosure.

- **Ethical guidelines and principles** play a crucial role in governing the ethical use of AI technologies in healthcare security. These guidelines provide a framework for ensuring that AI-driven solutions prioritize patient well-being, respect individual rights, uphold privacy and confidentiality, and promote fairness and transparency. By adhering to these ethical guidelines and principles, healthcare organizations can ensure that AI-driven security solutions uphold the highest ethical standards, protect patient rights, and promote trust, fairness, and transparency in healthcare delivery. Ethical considerations should be integrated into the design, development, deployment, and evaluation of AI technologies to ensure their responsible and ethical use in healthcare security (Fig. 7.6).

7.8.1 *Beneficence and Non-Maleficence*

- *Beneficence:* AI-enabled healthcare security solutions should aim to maximize benefits and improve patient outcomes. They should be designed to enhance the quality, safety, and efficiency of healthcare delivery while minimizing harm and mitigating risks.

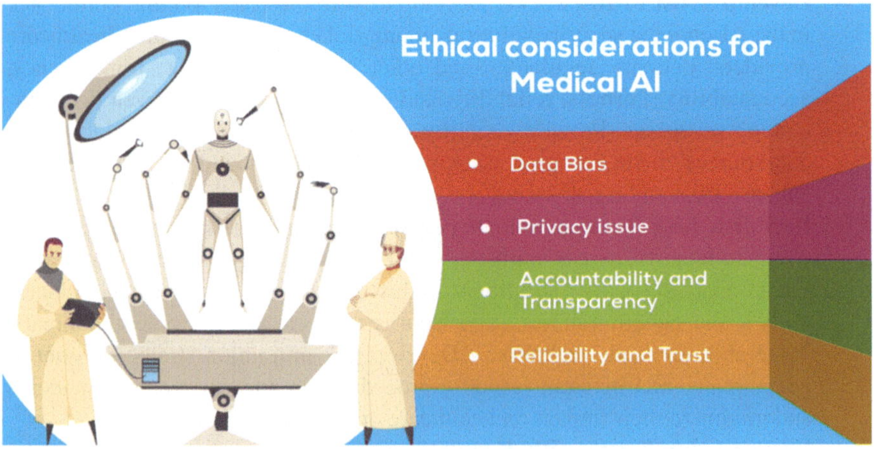

Fig. 7.6 Ethical considerations for Medical AI

- *Non-maleficence:* Healthcare organizations must ensure that AI technologies do not cause harm or pose risks to patients, healthcare providers, or other stakeholders. AI algorithms should be rigorously evaluated for potential adverse effects, unintended consequences, and biases that may result in harm to individuals.

7.8.2 Autonomy and Informed Consent

- *Autonomy*: Respect for patient autonomy is paramount in healthcare decision-making. AI-enabled security solutions should empower patients to make informed choices about their health information and treatment options. Patients should have control over the use and disclosure of their data and be able to exercise their rights to privacy and confidentiality.
- *Informed Consent:* Healthcare organizations should obtain informed consent from patients before using AI technologies to collect, process, or analyze their health data. Patients should be provided with clear and understandable information about the purpose, risks, benefits, and implications of AI-driven security solutions. They should have the opportunity to consent or withhold consent based on their preferences and values.

7.8.3 Privacy and Confidentiality

- *Privacy:* Protecting patient privacy is essential in AI-enabled healthcare security. Organizations must implement measures to safeguard the confidentiality of patient information and prevent unauthorized access, use, or disclosure. AI algorithms should adhere to privacy-preserving techniques such as data encryption, de-identification, and access controls to protect sensitive health data.
- *Confidentiality:* Healthcare organizations have a duty to maintain the confidentiality of patient information and protect it from unauthorized disclosure. AI technologies should be designed to ensure the secure storage, transmission, and processing of healthcare data, minimizing the risk of breaches or unauthorized access.

7.8.4 Fairness and Equity

- *Fairness*: AI algorithms should be designed and trained to promote fairness and equity in healthcare decision-making. Organizations must mitigate biases, discrimination, and disparities that may arise from the use of AI technologies, particularly in areas such as diagnosis, treatment, and resource allocation. They

should strive to ensure that AI-driven security solutions do not exacerbate existing inequalities or perpetuate unjust outcomes.
- *Equity:* Healthcare organizations should address disparities in access to healthcare services, resources, and technologies, including AI-enabled security solutions. They should ensure that AI technologies are accessible, inclusive, and equitable for all individuals, regardless of socioeconomic status, race, ethnicity, gender, or other factors.

7.8.5 Transparency and Explainability

- *Transparency:* Organizations should be transparent about the use of AI technologies in healthcare security and provide clear explanations of how AI algorithms work, what data they use, and how they make decisions. Transparency fosters trust, accountability, and understanding among stakeholders, including patients, healthcare providers, regulators, and the public.
- *Explainability*: AI-driven security solutions should be designed to be explainable and interpretable, enabling stakeholders to understand the rationale behind AI-driven decisions and actions. Organizations should provide insights into the underlying logic, factors, and considerations that inform AI algorithms' recommendations or predictions. Explainability helps build confidence in AI technologies and enables stakeholders to assess their reliability, accuracy, and fairness.

7.8.6 Accountability and Responsibility

- *Accountability:* Healthcare organizations are accountable for the ethical use of AI technologies in healthcare security. They must establish mechanisms for accountability, oversight, and compliance with ethical guidelines and regulatory requirements. Organizations should monitor the performance, impact, and outcomes of AI-driven security solutions and take responsibility for addressing any ethical concerns or violations that may arise.
- *Responsibility:* Healthcare professionals, data scientists, developers, and other stakeholders involved in the development and deployment of AI technologies have a responsibility to uphold ethical standards and prioritize patient welfare. They should adhere to ethical codes of conduct, professional guidelines, and best practices for responsible AI development and use in healthcare security.

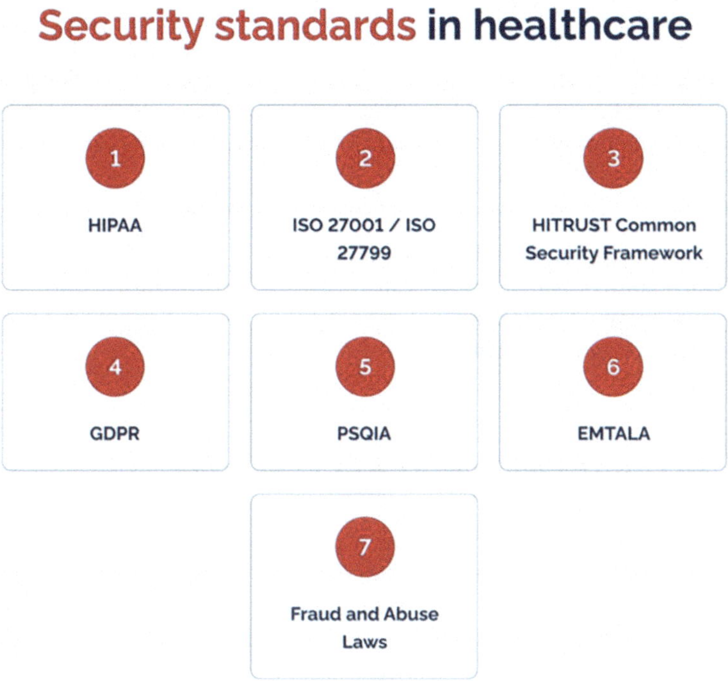
Security standards in healthcare
1
HIPAA
2
ISO 27001 / ISO 27799
3
HITRUST Common Security Framework
4
GDPR
5
PSQIA
6
EMTALA
7
Fraud and Abuse Laws

Fig. 7.7 Healthcare standards

7.9 Healthcare Data Security Standards (Fig. 7.7)

7.9.1 HIPAA

The Health Insurance Portability and Accountability Act improves accountability and health insurance coverage. At first, the government tried to systematize medical patient records and initiated the HIPAA privacy regulations and social security rules [15, 16].

HIPAA regulations provide a set of security standards that healthcare entities must adhere to:

1. HIPAA Privacy Rule;
2. HIPAA Security Rule;
3. HIPAA Enforcement Rule;
4. HIPAA Breach Notification Rule.

However, there is no clear list of approved security solutions, technology providers, or HIPAA-compliant software pieces.

7.9.2 ISO 27001/ISO 27799

To protect confidential medical information, two necessary international security standards should be applied. ISO 27001 sets clear requirements for an information security management system. Whereas ISO 27799 provides best practices for working with data flow in healthcare [15].

In turn, ISO 27799 is threatened by the following problems in particular:

- Illegal use of a program with health information;
- Implementation of malicious software;
- Communication interception;
- Operator, user, or maintenance error.

7.9.3 HITRUST Common Security Framework

HITRUST CSF is a global framework that meets security standards to ensure ISO and HIPAA requirements. Covered entities can quickly respond to audit requests for health data security standards, saving buyer and supplier time and resources.

There are also other essential healthcare data security standards:

7.9.4 GDPR

The General Data Protection Regulation provides new rules for processing website users' personal data. In particular, the restrictions apply to EU citizens, even if these sites are located outside the EU but are used by these residents. Then it's necessary to optimize your services and areas according to the requirements of the GDPR regarding security, for example, credit card data, profile data when registering at a hotel, and passport data of users [15].

To implement GDPR in your company, requires to check the affiliation of customers and partners to the EU. Then one can proceed to the implementation of changes under GDPR requirements. Next, one should assess the risks of late change implementation and use tools that will to adapt to the new conditions of service provision.

7.9.5 PSQIA

The Patient Safety and Quality Improvement Act provides a reporting system to improve health data security and address patient safety and care quality. The Act also guarantees the confidentiality of patient safety information, authorizing HHS to impose civil monetary penalties for violations of patient confidentiality. The Act also coordinates the Agency for Healthcare Research and Quality's listing of Patient Safety Organizations (PSOs) [15].

7.9.6 EMTALA

The Emergency Medical Treatment and Labor Act provides stabilization and treatment regardless of patients' insurance status or ability to pay. Since 1986, the law has lost its mandate and state funding, so emergency physicians provide the most charitable care of any physician.

EMTALA requires emergency hospitals to evaluate and treat emergency medical conditions of patients without regard to nationality, race, or financial status [15].

7.9.7 Fraud and Abuse Laws

National laws prohibiting fraud and abuse of office also apply to health care providers. Medical professionals are prohibited from providing false invoices to private or public insurance companies or prescribing unnecessary drugs for personal enrichment. Money laundering by employees through medical institutions is also severely punished.

Local laws can vary greatly. Health care organizations need to be aware of local legal requirements and ensure that their systems comply strictly to prevent problems with law enforcement.

7.10 Ensuring Data Privacy and Security

1. **Implement Data Encryption:** Implement encryption techniques to protect sensitive healthcare data both in transit and at rest. Encrypt data using strong cryptographic algorithms and secure key management practices to prevent unauthorized access or interception. Use encryption protocols such as Transport Layer Security (TLS) for securing data in transit and encryption algorithms such as Advanced Encryption Standard (AES) for securing data at rest. Use strong encryption algorithms to safeguard sensitive medical information. Encryption ensures that even if unwanted access happens, the data is rendered unreadable and unusable.
2. **Enforce Access Controls:** Enforce strict access controls to limit access to patient data and sensitive information. Implement role-based access controls (RBAC), attribute-based access controls (ABAC), and least privilege principles to restrict access to authorized users based on their roles, responsibilities, and

permissions. Use authentication mechanisms such as passwords, biometric authentication, multi-factor authentication (MFA), and single sign-on (SSO) to verify the identity of users and ensure secure access to healthcare systems and applications.

3. **Monitor and Audit User Activities:** Implement monitoring and auditing mechanisms to track and record user activities, system events, and security incidents. Monitor user logins, access attempts, data accesses, file transfers, and other activities to detect suspicious behavior, unauthorized access, or security breaches. Use security information and event management (SIEM) systems, intrusion detection systems (IDS), and log management tools to collect, analyze, and correlate security logs and events for threat detection, incident response, and forensic analysis. Use AI-powered surveillance equipment to spot suspicious activity or patterns in real time. These technologies can detect potential safety violations and notify the appropriate authorities for rapid action.
4. **Regularly Update and Patch Systems:** Regularly update and patch healthcare systems, software applications, operating systems, and firmware to address known vulnerabilities, security flaws, and software bugs. Keep abreast of security advisories, alerts, and patches released by vendors, manufacturers, and cybersecurity organizations. Establish patch management processes, change control procedures, and vulnerability management programs to ensure timely deployment of security updates and patches across all systems and devices.
5. **Frequent Security Audits:** Execute frequent security audits to discover system vulnerabilities and shortcomings. These audits assist in discovering and responding to possible threats or breaches in the shortest possible time.
6. **Secure Data Storage:** Medical data should be stored in secure, encrypted systems. Implement access restrictions and strong authentication methods to ensure that sensitive information is only accessed by authorized persons.

7.11 Best Practices for Protecting Healthcare Data

There are various best practices for protecting healthcare data. Figure 7.8 shows four best practices.

7.11.1 Improving the Quality of Medical Personnel

Improving the quality of medical personnel develops the ability to implement the received training into action. Enhancing the knowledge of healthcare workers should include skills in managing complexity, leading change, and reflection. In training, they will also become resilient to the human factors that affect patient capacity and engagement throughout the process [17].

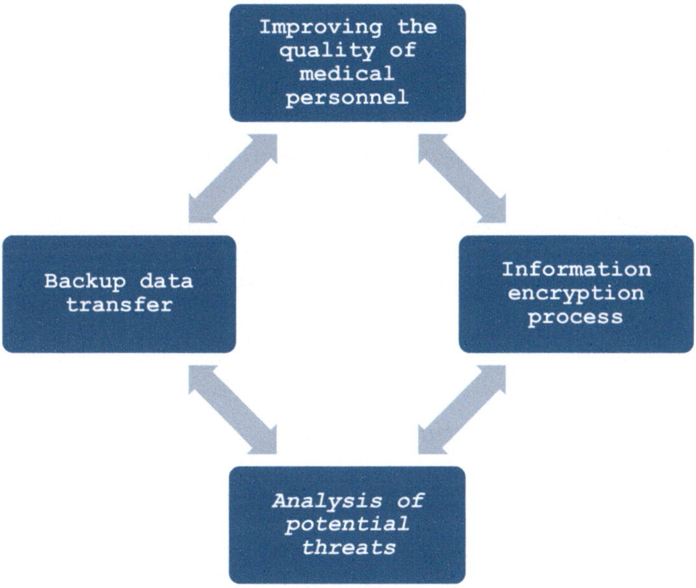

Fig. 7.8 Best practices for protecting healthcare data

Healthcare professionals should be trained to understand the importance of health data security, recognize phishing attempts, identify hazardous web pages or files, clean the computer system, and act appropriately in case of a system error. Healthcare organizations should conduct regular training sessions and workshops to ensure that all employees are on the same page, know how vital patient data loss prevention measures are, and are devoted to the organization [18].

7.11.2 Information Encryption Process

Encrypting information is an important preventive step to restrain hackers from decoding it. The development team develops the most suitable method for individual platforms—symmetric or asymmetric access key. You can encrypt your private network with Virtual Private Network without being an expert. Then outside the private network, it's challenging to identify the data and upload or download it from your personal computer. Secure Hypertext Transfer Protocol, Secure File Transfer Protocol, and Secure Sockets Layer also ensure private data security.

Benefits of encrypting medical data:

- Data protection when the user uses different types of devices;
- Combination with advanced authentication to make data more secure;
- Prevention of material losses due to data leakage.

For example, your company can be punished with significant fines if attackers get access to confidential information.

It's also worth considering some practices that will help you effectively encrypt medical data:

1. Regularly assess security risks to identify when encryption is proper.
2. Minimization of costs to prevent large-scale modification of the existing IT infrastructure.
3. Key management to ensure the future recovery of encrypted data.
4. Ability to encrypt data on all removable media and external devices to protect PHI.

7.11.3 Analysis of Potential Threats

There are threats in every practice, but too many people or institutions ignore or minimize healthcare data security challenges. The best way to identify threats is to form a SWOT analysis based on competitor research and subsequent priorities. Threats can haunt a medical facility from anywhere, including:

- unfavorable conditions in compensation or rules.
- loss of key personnel or partners.
- changes in market demand or recommendations.

7.11.4 Backup Data Transfer

Knowing how to store medical records and choosing a good backup strategy is necessary. Ensuring high standards of data integrity and access is an important task for healthcare providers. The vulnerable healthcare system requires an extremely secure backup. Therefore, it's imperative for healthcare organizations to assess their security requirements and take appropriate measures to implement strong data protection.

The most proven and reliable method of protecting medical data remains the 3-2-1 Backup Strategy. It guarantees at least three copies of your data on two different devices and at least one in the cloud. If you back up your NAS device to cloud storage, this will be the third external copy.

IBackup also provides a backup and storage solution for the security and protection of critical data without compromising patient privacy. The program securely archives all information and prevents illegal access by storing data in encrypted form [19].

7.11.4.1 Who to Trust in Data Security in Healthcare?

Health Organizations must choose technical experts who follow transparent and ethical approach in their medical software development services. The healthcare organizations need to have medical and technical expertsso as to develop the healthcare app or a web based secure platform to maintain patient healthcare information.

7.12 Conclusion

In conclusion, the integration of Artificial Intelligence (AI) into healthcare systems has brought about transformative advancements in patient care, diagnosis, treatment, and administrative processes. However, these remarkable achievements are accompanied by significant concerns regarding the security and privacy of patient information. As healthcare organizations collect vast amounts of sensitive data, they become prime targets for cyber-attacks.

It is imperative that we comprehend the landscape of AI-enabled healthcare security to safeguard patient information and uphold the integrity of our health systems. To achieve this, robust security solutions are paramount. AI-enabled healthcare security systems offer critical measures to protect patient data and instill trust in the healthcare system.

This chapter has delved into the best practices for designing and implementing AI-enabled healthcare security solutions. These practices include the integration of existing systems, the establishment of governance and trust frameworks, and the assurance of data privacy and security. By adhering to these best practices, healthcare organizations can effectively mitigate security risks, safeguard patient information, and maintain the integrity and confidentiality of healthcare systems and data.

In addition to these practices, it is essential to highlight some key aspects of healthcare security solutions. Firstly, continuous monitoring and analysis of network traffic using AI algorithms enable early detection and prevention of cyber threats. Secondly, anomaly detection and predictive analytics play a pivotal role in identifying potential security issues before they escalate into breaches. Lastly, access control mechanisms powered by AI help in ensuring that only authorized personnel have access to sensitive patient data.

By embracing these healthcare security solutions and best practices, healthcare organizations can fortify their defenses against cyber threats, thereby safeguarding patient information and upholding trust in the healthcare system. As we continue to navigate the ever-evolving landscape of AI-enabled healthcare, prioritizing security remains essential to ensure the well-being of patients and the integrity of healthcare systems.

References

1. Kocabas, O. E., & Aktas, H. (2020). A secure and efficient patient information system with attribute-based encryption in cloud-based e-healthcare applications. Future Generation Computer Systems, 102, 467–477.
2. https://keenethics.com/blog/healthcare-data-security
3. Wang, Y., Kung, L., & Byrd, T. A. (2018). Big data analytics: Understanding its capabilities and potential benefits for healthcare organizations. Technological Forecasting and Social Change, 126, 3–13.
4. Williams, P. A. H., Woodward, A. J., & Goel, S. (2020). Effects of phishing awareness training on reducing successful phishing attacks in healthcare organizations. Computers & Security, 95, 101834.
5. Fruhlinger, J. (2022). WannaCry explained: A perfect ransomware storm. CSO Online.
6. Indian healthcare industry sees second highest number of cyber attacks in the world: CloudSEK. (2022, September 20). The Economic Times. https://economictimes.indiatimes.com/industry/healthcare/biotech/healthcare/indian-healthcare-industry-sees-second-highest-number-of-cyber-attacks-in-the-world-cloudsek/articleshow/94327718.cms
7. Cyberattack Paralyzes the Largest U.S. Health Care Payment System. (2024, March 5). https://www.nytimes.com/2024/03/05/health/cyberattack-healthcare-cash.html
8. Shortliffe, E. H., & Sepúlveda, M. J. (2018). Clinical decision support in the era of artificial intelligence. JAMA, 320(21), 2199–2200.
9. Bajwa, J., Munir, U., Nori, A., & Williams, B. (2021). Artificial intelligence in healthcare: transforming the practice of medicine. Future healthcare journal, 8(2), e188.
10. Nijhawan, R., Ansari, S. A., Kumar, S., Alassery, F., & El-Kenawy, S. M. (2022). Gun identification from gunshot audios for secure public places using transformer learning. Scientific reports, 12(1), 13300.
11. Imoize, A. L., Balas, V. E., Solanki, V. K., Lee, C. C., & Obaidat, M. S. (Eds.). (2023). Handbook of Security and Privacy of AI-Enabled Healthcare Systems and Internet of Medical Things. CRC Press.
12. Chatterjee, S., & Pal, S. (2020). Cybersecurity in healthcare: A systematic review of trends and challenges. Computers & Security, 88, 101682.
13. Pandey, F., Gupta, S., & Kumar, S. (2014). Information hiding using image steganography-A survey. Journal of Basic and Applied Engineering Research (JBAER), 14, 854.
14. Lee, J., & Kim, J. (2019). Governance for Healthcare Security in the Age of Artificial Intelligence. Journal of Healthcare Information Management, 33(2), 18–24.
15. Tang, P. C., & Machiraju, R. (2017). Standards and interoperability in healthcare information systems: Current state and future challenges. In Healthcare Information Management Systems (pp. 3–22). Springer, Cham.
16. Chithaluru, P., Singh, A., Mahmoud, M. S., Kumar, S., Mazón, J. L. V., Alkhayyat, A., & Anand, D. (2023). An enhanced opportunistic rank-based parent node selection for sustainable & smart IoT networks. Sustainable Energy Technologies and Assessments, 56, 103079.
17. Kawamoto, K. (2016). Healthcare information management systems: Cases, strategies, and solutions. Springer.
18. Chen, C., & Zheng, L. (2018). Information security and privacy: A practical guide for global executives, lawyers and technologists. Wiley.
19. Choi, D. M., & Chung, K. J. (2019). Securing the Internet of Medical Things: Challenges, threats, and security solutions. Health Information Science and Systems, 7(1), 1–11.

Chapter 8
Impact of AI-Enabled Healthcare Security on Patient Outcomes

Contents

Abstract The advancements promised by AI enabled healthcare have inherent vulnerability aspects concerning patient privacy and adoption of timely cybersecurity measures to protect sensitive healthcare data. AI algorithms for threat detection, anomaly detection, and predictive analytics, healthcare organisations are very useful in identification and mitigation of security threats. This results in least disruption in patient care regime and therefore ensures the confidentiality of patient information. This chapter is aimed to provide discussions on potential impact of AI-enabled healthcare security on patient outcomes. The chapter also provides insights into good case studies of hospitals and organizations who have successfully deployed AI to manage patient centric AI-enabled healthcare security solutions.

Keywords Healthcare security · Artificial intelligence · Risk identification · Risk mitigation · Cybersecurity

S. Gupta et al., *Artificial Intelligence-Enabled Security for Healthcare Systems*,
https://doi.org/10.1007/978-3-031-82810-2_8

8.1 Introduction

In a time when technology is developing at an exponential rate, the way medical services are structured, managed, and optimized is changing dramatically in the healthcare sector. The integration of cutting-edge modern technologies is the primary motivating factor behind this change, with artificial intelligence (AI) emerging as a revolutionary force that has the ability to drastically alter healthcare as it exists now. AI's importance becomes evident as medical professionals and agencies work to deliver more precise diagnosis, customized treatment regimens, and efficient managerial procedures. AI has begun to play an increasingly important part in healthcare, from researching novel medications to managing medical tasks and assisting doctors with diagnosis. AI methods, such as machine learning and deep learning, may sift through enormous quantities of healthcare information in order to identify trends and make predictions [1]. Figure 8.1 shows the impact of AI in healthcare.

AI, for instance, can assist medical professionals in identifying issues in imaging data, enabling quicker and more precise diagnoses. According to Frost and Sullivan's predictions, using AI is expected to save treatment costs by 50% while also enhancing patient outcomes. While it comes to determining the diagnosis and outlook of diseases, AI models can analyze enormous quantities of patient data, including symptoms, medical history, and genetic data. The development of more accurate and effective disease diagnosis is facilitated by this approach. Artificial intelligence algorithms can recognize patterns that human doctors might find challenging to recognize, and this results in earlier detection and better accuracy. Because AI is capable of analyzing enormous datasets and discovering promising drug candidates, it holds promise for speeding up the drug discovery process [2].

Molecular structures can be analyzed and predictions about the efficacy and possible negative effects of medications can be made by utilizing machine learning techniques. The discovery and development of novel cures and treatments may proceed more quickly and affordably as a result of this expedited drug candidate

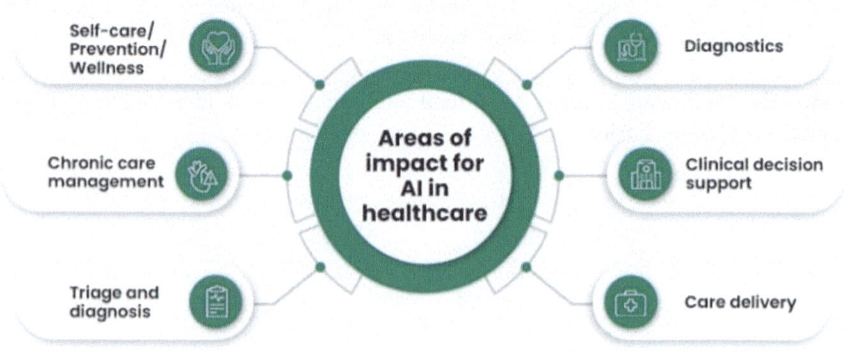
Self-care/
Prevention/
Wellness
Diagnostics
Areas of
impact for
AI in
healthcare
Chronic care
management
Clinical decision
support
Triage and
diagnosis
Care delivery

Fig. 8.1 Impact of AI in healthcare [1]

screening procedure. An increasing number of people are using chatbots and virtual assistants powered by artificial intelligence (AI) to evaluate symptoms, answer patient questions, and provide basic medical information. They are essential in helping with medicine reminders, appointment scheduling, and following treatment monitoring. These AI-powered solutions improve the satisfaction of patients and accessibility to healthcare, which makes the patient experience more seamless [3].

The way medical practitioners monitor patients' well-being has been completely transformed by AI-driven patient monitoring. Vital indications including heart rate, blood pressure, and oxygen levels are continuously collected and analyzed by wearable technology and AI-powered remote monitoring systems. The aforementioned technologies can automatically notify nurses and other healthcare personnel when anomalies or alarming trends are found, enabling prompt responses. Patients recovering from surgery or those with chronic diseases benefit most from this real-time monitoring capacity since it allows for early intervention and lessens the need for ongoing in-person supervision. Nurses can improve patient outcomes and care quality by more effectively allocating their time and concentrating on patients who need immediate treatment [4].

8.2 AI-Driven Advancements in Patient Care and Treatment

Figure 8.2 shows the AI applications in healthcare. AI-driven advancements in patient care and treatment have revolutionized healthcare delivery by enhancing diagnostic accuracy, personalizing treatment plans, improving patient outcomes, and optimizing healthcare workflows [5].

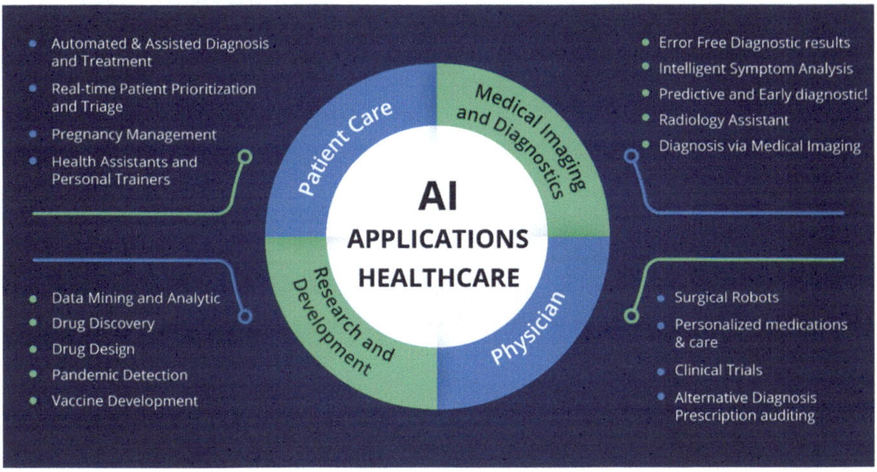

Fig. 8.2 AI applications in healthcare [5]

I. **Medical Imaging Interpretation**: AI algorithms can analyze medical images, such as X-rays, MRI scans, and CT scans, with remarkable accuracy. These algorithms can detect abnormalities, lesions, and other indicators of disease, assisting radiologists in diagnosing conditions like cancer, fractures, and neurological disorders more quickly and accurately. For instance, AI-based systems like Google's DeepMind Health and IBM Watson Health can identify patterns and anomalies in medical images, aiding radiologists in interpretation and diagnosis. Figure 8.3 shows the medical imaging interpretation.

II. **Predictive Analytics for Disease Prevention**: AI models can analyze large datasets of patient health records, genetic information, and lifestyle factors to predict an individual's risk of developing certain diseases or health complications. By identifying high-risk patients, healthcare providers can intervene early with preventive measures, such as lifestyle modifications, regular screenings, or targeted interventions. For example, AI-driven predictive analytics tools can forecast the risk of cardiovascular disease, diabetes, or sepsis, enabling proactive management and prevention strategies.

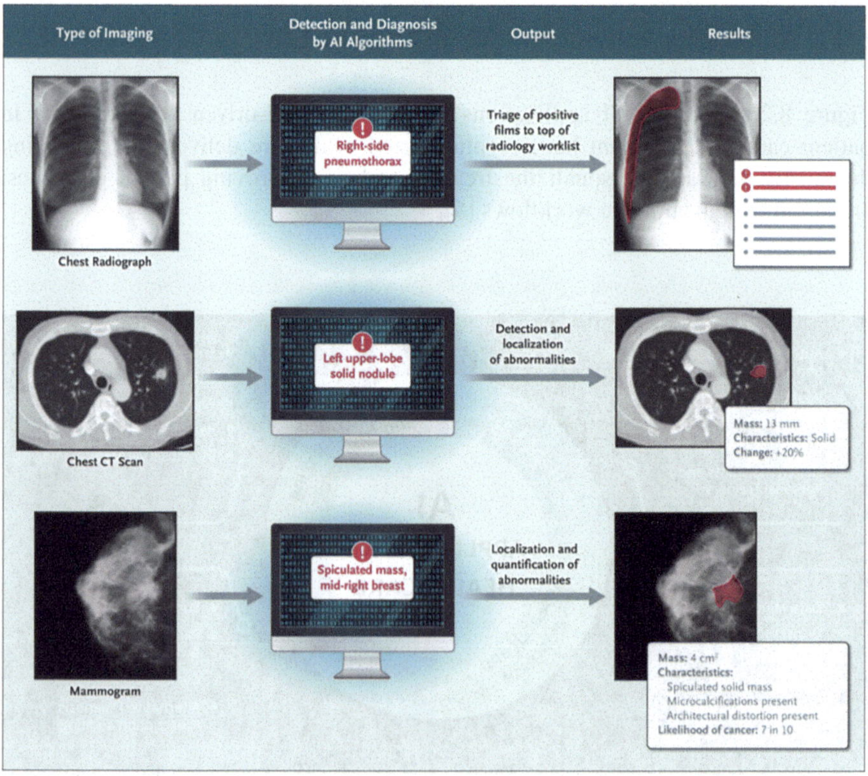

Fig. 8.3 Medical imaging interpretation [6]

III. **Precision Medicine and Personalized Treatment**: AI enables the development of personalized treatment plans tailored to an individual's unique genetic makeup, medical history, and disease characteristics. By analyzing genomic data, biomarkers, and treatment responses, AI algorithms can identify the most effective therapies and predict patient responses to specific medications. This approach, known as precision medicine, maximizes treatment efficacy while minimizing adverse effects. Companies like Tempus and Foundation Medicine utilize AI to analyze genomic data and guide personalized cancer treatment decisions. Figure 8.4 depicts the precision medicine and personalized treatment [7].

IV. **Virtual Health Assistants and Remote Monitoring**: AI-powered virtual health assistants, chatbots, and telehealth platforms enable remote patient monitoring, symptom assessment, and personalized health guidance. These digital health tools can provide 24/7 access to healthcare information, answer patient queries, and offer real-time support for managing chronic conditions or post-operative care. For example, Babylon Health's AI chatbot assists patients in triaging symptoms and accessing healthcare services remotely,

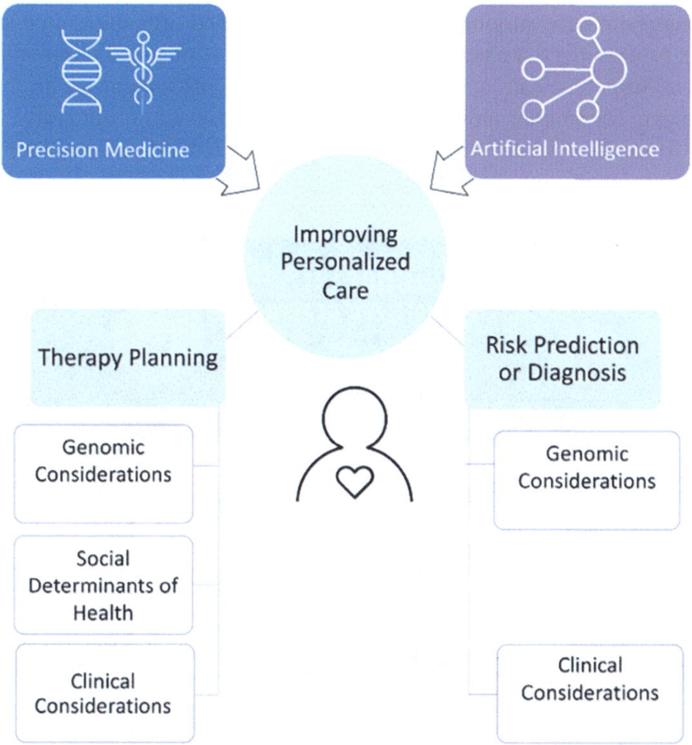

Fig. 8.4 Precision medicine and personalized treatment [7]

improving access to care and reducing unnecessary hospital visits. Figure 8.5 shows a chatbot for virtual health assistant.

V. **Drug Discovery and Development**: AI accelerates the drug discovery process by analyzing large-scale biological datasets, identifying potential drug targets, and predicting drug efficacy and safety profiles. Machine learning algorithms can sift through vast amounts of chemical and biological data to discover novel drug candidates, optimize drug design, and repurpose existing medications for new therapeutic applications. Companies like Insilico Medicine and Atomwise leverage AI for drug discovery, shortening the time and cost required to bring new treatments to market.

VI. **Clinical Decision Support Systems**: AI-powered clinical decision support systems integrate with electronic health records (EHRs) to provide evidence-based recommendations for diagnosis, treatment planning, and medication management. These systems analyze patient data, medical literature, and clinical guidelines to assist healthcare providers in making informed decisions at the point of care. By offering personalized treatment suggestions and alerting clinicians to potential risks or contraindications, AI-driven decision support systems improve care quality, reduce medical errors, and enhance patient safety.

VII. **Robotic Surgery and Minimally Invasive Procedures**: AI-enabled robotic systems enhance surgical precision, dexterity, and efficiency, enabling complex procedures to be performed with greater accuracy and minimal invasiveness. Surgeons can control robotic surgical instruments with precision, allowing for smaller incisions, reduced blood loss, and faster recovery times. Platforms like the da Vinci Surgical System utilize AI and machine learning

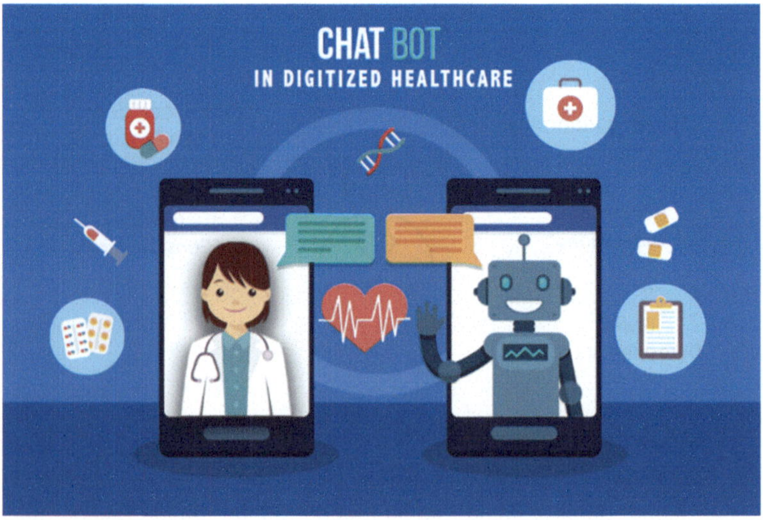

Fig. 8.5 Virtual health assistant

algorithms to assist surgeons in performing minimally invasive surgeries across various specialties, including urology, gynecology, and cardiothoracic surgery. Figure 8.6 shows the process of robot assisted surgery.

VIII. **Patient data protection:** The utilization of AI in healthcare heavily depends on access to patient data, including medical records, diagnostic images, and genetic information. While AI can potentially improve patient care and outcomes, it also raises significant concerns about data privacy. Safeguarding sensitive health information is crucial to maintaining patient trust and complying with healthcare regulations like HIPAA (Health Insurance Portability and Accountability Act). Robust security measures, such as encryption, access controls, and auditing, are essential to protect patient data from unauthorized access or breaches. Ethical data handling and adherence to stringent privacy regulations are fundamental to ensure that AI-driven healthcare remains safe and respectful of patient privacy.

IX. **Data breaches:** The interconnected nature of healthcare systems, along with the growing reliance on electronic health records, makes the healthcare sector particularly vulnerable to cyberattacks and data breaches. Data breaches can compromise patient privacy and safety, as well as erode public trust in healthcare providers. The consequences of such breaches can be severe, leading to identity theft, fraudulent medical claims, and even incorrect medical treatments. Robust cybersecurity measures, regular system updates, and staff training are essential to mitigate these risks and ensure the security of patient data in an AI-driven healthcare environment. Healthcare organizations must

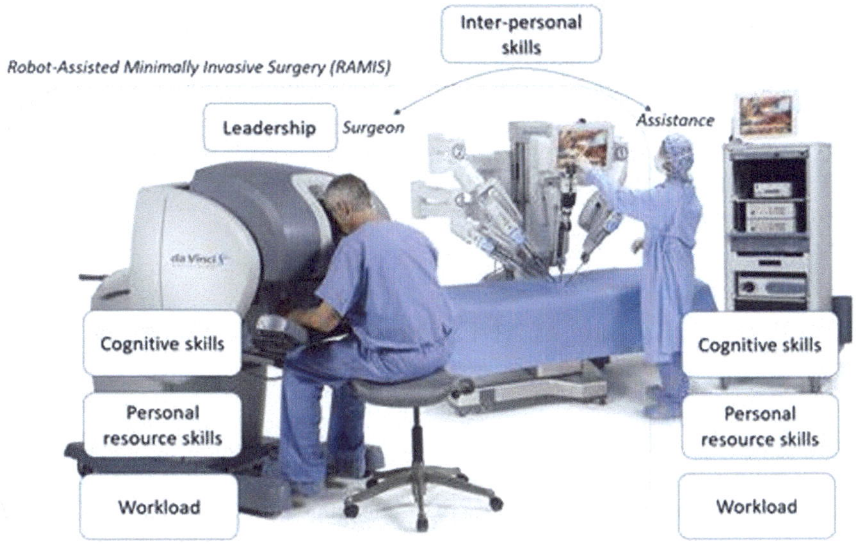

Fig. 8.6 Robot assisted surgery [7]

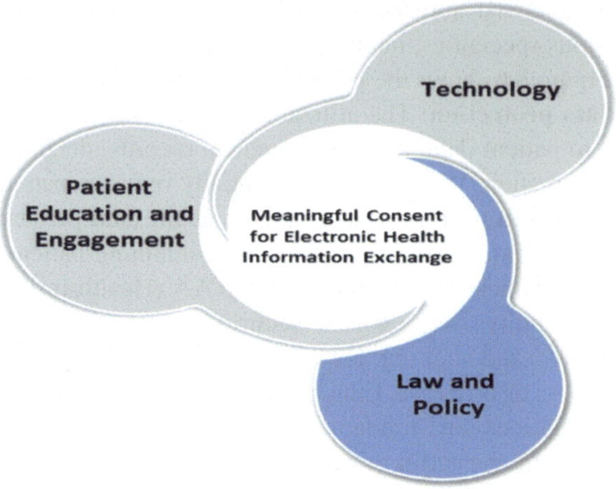

Fig. 8.7 Patient data security [7]

also have well-defined incident response plans to address breaches promptly and minimize their impact.

X. **Informed consent:** The use of AI in healthcare requires patients to provide informed consent, indicating that they understand the implications of AI-driven care. However, ensuring that patients fully comprehend the intricacies of AI can be challenging. AI systems often involve complex algorithms and large datasets that may need to be explained to patients. To address this, healthcare providers and organizations must invest in patient education and transparent communication. They should inform patients about the role of AI in their care, its potential benefits, and the safeguards in place to protect their data. Providing patients with clear and accessible information is essential to obtaining informed consent and respecting patient autonomy while incorporating AI into healthcare practices. Patients must have confidence in AI systems and trust that their data will be handled securely and ethically. Figure 8.7 shows the patient data security.

8.3 Potential Impact of AI-Enabled Healthcare Security on Patient Outcomes

AI-enabled healthcare security has the potential to revolutionize patient care by enhancing data security, enabling preventive interventions, streamlining diagnosis and treatment planning, and providing real-time clinical decision support. By leveraging AI technologies to safeguard patient data and optimize healthcare delivery, organizations can achieve better patient outcomes, improve care quality, and

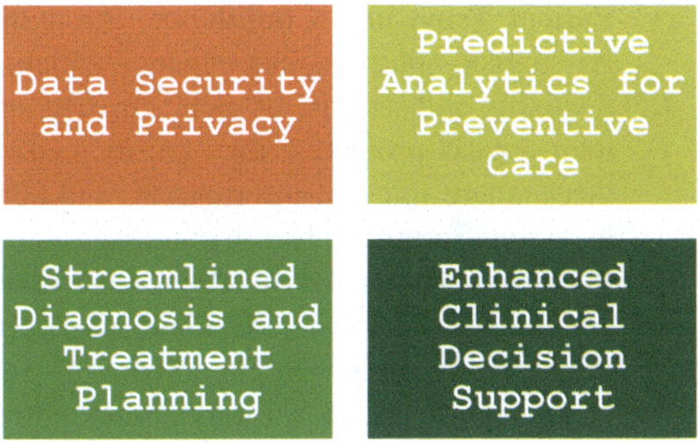

Fig. 8.8 AI-enabled healthcare security on patient outcomes

enhance overall patient experience [6–9]. Figure 8.8 shows AI-enabled healthcare security on patient outcomes. The potential impact of AI-enabled healthcare security on patient outcomes is significant and multifaceted. Here are several key points outlining this potential impact:

(i) **Data Security and Privacy**: AI can enhance data security by continuously monitoring and identifying potential threats to patient data. By implementing advanced encryption techniques and anomaly detection algorithms, AI can safeguard patient information from unauthorized access, breaches, or cyber-attacks. Enhanced data security and privacy measures instil trust among patients, encouraging them to share sensitive health information more freely with healthcare providers. This facilitates better diagnosis and treatment planning, ultimately leading to improved patient outcomes.AI-driven security solutions can detect and mitigate security threats more effectively than traditional methods, reducing the risk of data breaches and unauthorized access to patient information. This enhances patient privacy and safeguards sensitive healthcare data.

(ii) **Improved Care Delivery:** By streamlining administrative processes, optimizing resource allocation, and enhancing operational efficiency, AI-enabled security measures enable healthcare providers to focus more on patient care. This can lead to improved care delivery, timely interventions, and better patient outcomes.

(iii) **Early Detection of Security Threats:** AI algorithms can analyze large volumes of data in real-time to identify anomalies and potential security threats. By detecting threats early, healthcare organizations can take proactive measures to mitigate risks, minimize disruptions to patient care, and ensure continuity of services.

(iv) **Proactive Risk Management:** AI-driven predictive analytics can forecast potential security threats and vulnerabilities based on historical data and trends. By identifying emerging risks, healthcare organizations can implement proactive security measures to prevent data breaches, protect patient information, and maintain the integrity of healthcare systems.

(v) **Patient Trust and Confidence**: Strengthening healthcare security through AI-enabled solutions can enhance patient trust and confidence in the confidentiality and security of their sensitive information. When patients trust that their data is protected, they are more likely to engage with healthcare services, share relevant information, and adhere to treatment plans, ultimately leading to improved health outcomes.

(vi) **Predictive Analytics for Preventive Care**: AI algorithms can analyze vast amounts of patient data to identify patterns and trends that human analysts might miss. By leveraging predictive analytics, AI can forecast potential health risks or diseases in individual patients, allowing healthcare providers to intervene early with preventive measures. For example, AI can analyze patient data to identify individuals at high risk of developing chronic conditions like diabetes or cardiovascular disease, enabling healthcare professionals to implement targeted interventions such as lifestyle modifications or early screenings. By focusing on preventive care, AI-enabled healthcare security can help reduce the incidence of severe health complications, leading to better patient outcomes and lower healthcare costs.

(vii) **Streamlined Diagnosis and Treatment Planning**: AI-powered diagnostic tools can assist healthcare providers in accurately diagnosing medical conditions and developing personalized treatment plans. Machine learning algorithms trained on vast datasets of medical images, patient records, and clinical guidelines can help radiologists and clinicians interpret diagnostic tests more efficiently and accurately. Additionally, AI can analyze genetic data to identify biomarkers associated with specific diseases, enabling precision medicine approaches tailored to individual patients. By streamlining the diagnostic process and facilitating personalized treatment strategies, AI-enabled healthcare security can improve patient outcomes by reducing misdiagnosis rates, optimizing treatment efficacy, and minimizing adverse effects.

(viii) **Enhanced Clinical Decision Support**: AI can provide real-time clinical decision support to healthcare providers at the point of care. By integrating with electronic health record (EHR) systems and analysing patient data in real-time, AI algorithms can offer evidence-based recommendations for diagnosis, treatment, and medication management. For instance, AI-powered clinical decision support systems can alert clinicians to potential drug interactions, suggest appropriate dosage adjustments based on patient-specific factors, or recommend alternative treatment options supported by the latest medical research. By augmenting clinical decision-making with AI-driven insights, healthcare providers can make more informed choices that align with best practices and patient preferences, leading to better treatment outcomes and improved patient satisfaction.

8.3.1 *Guarding Patient Privacy: The Healthcare Cybersecurity `Dilemma*

The healthcare sector's transition to a digitally driven environment has brought about numerous benefits, but it has also introduced a host of cybersecurity challenges. Below are the challenges of implementing cybersecurity with vivid examples, by understanding these challenges and learning from past incidents, healthcare organizations can take proactive measures to bolster their cybersecurity defences and ensure the safety and privacy of both patient data and critical medical operations [10].

(i) **Resource constraints and budget limitations:** Many smaller healthcare providers often struggle with limited budgets and resources for cybersecurity initiatives. This can result in delayed updates, insufficient training for staff, and a lack of investment in advanced cybersecurity tools. Such challenges make them attractive targets for cybercriminals.

(ii) **Human error and insider threats:** A simple error, like an employee accidentally sending patient data to the wrong email address, can lead to significant breaches. Additionally, malicious insider threats can exploit their access for personal gain. The case of a hospital employee selling patient data to identity thieves serves as a poignant reminder of the risks associated with human fallibility and malicious intent.

(iii) **Interconnected systems and third-party risks:** The NotPetya malware attack in 2017 significantly affected operations at various healthcare facilities by targeting a third-party Ukrainian accounting software. This incident highlighted the potential consequences of interconnected systems and the cascading effects of a cyberattack on a seemingly unrelated service provider [11].

(iv) **Medical device vulnerabilities**: The vulnerabilities in medical devices came to the forefront with the case of the Medtronic insulin pump hack. Researchers found that the device could be remotely manipulated, potentially leading to incorrect insulin doses being administered, risking patient safety and raising concerns about the security of Internet of Things (IoT) devices in healthcare.

(v) **Data breaches and patient privacy violations**: In 2015, Anthem Inc., one of the largest health insurance companies in the US, fell victim to a massive data breach where the personal information of nearly 78.8 million customers was compromised. The breach exposed sensitive data including names, addresses, and Social Security numbers, highlighting the grave consequences of inadequate cybersecurity measures.

The AI system, though designed to improve patient care, becomes a vulnerability if not fortified with robust cybersecurity measures. The incidents highlight the urgent need for future healthcare leaders to integrate AI and cybersecurity seamlessly. While facing the challenges posed by AI and cybersecurity, a clarion call goes out to future healthcare leaders who possess the vision, knowledge, and determination to drive positive change. These leaders must champion the integration of AI while maintaining an unwavering commitment to cybersecurity.

8.3.2 Strengthening Cybersecurity Measures in Healthcare

Be it healthcare or any other sector, cybersecurity is important for continuity of business. It's more important in healthcare as it deals with patients' safety and treatment. Compromise on digital infrastructure of a healthcare entity is graver than anything else. Steps need to be taken for ensuring the digital environment is secure and safe for use. These steps do not need to be taken at some select levels. Security needs to be strengthened at all levels right from the entry point, i.e. the Firewall, to the end users compute device security like access and USB ports blocking [12].

- The initial steps in this direction start at the very top, i.e., at the end user level. Access to any kind of data and application should be only through a well-defined approval matrix and should be clearly documented. All access control should be role based. No access should be given without proper approval hierarchy being followed.
- Post approval, logging in to any application must be through multifactor authentication.
- USB ports and access to internet must not be allowed unless very important. If any of these things need to be allowed, it should be done securely in a different network thus maintaining sanctity of the main network.
- These days with the prevalence of online platforms like Microsoft OneDrive and Google Drive, the use for pen drives has gone down significantly. These online drives allow users to store their data to a cloud with already in place tight security and at the same time allows them to access this data from anywhere thus eliminating the dependency on the devices and presence before the device to share the data. Users can share data from these online drives from any device (desktop, laptop or smartphone) to anyone and anywhere in the entire world.

Patient data stored on servers and data storage devices is the most critical and most important class of patient data in any healthcare organization. Therefore, it becomes pertinent that not just security, but availability of this data is maintained round the clock all through the year [13].

- Such data whether it be a database, medical images or scanned documents, should be in an encrypted format, so that, even if any external entity gets to this data, should not be able to access or re-encrypt it.
- This data should be stored at two locations that are independent of each other. It is important that a real-time copy of the production data should be maintained at a far-off remote location.

This is called **Disaster Recovery (DR)** or **Business Continuity Process (BCP)**. Let us for a moment assume, that an external entity gets through the firewalls, access the data and then encrypts it too. At this time, the data becomes inaccessible for the organization thus putting the entire set of operations dependent on this data to come to a standstill. At this time, if there is a real time copy of this data available at any other secure location, the business can easily continue their processes from this location.

8.3.3 Improved Care Delivery with Patient Data Security and Outcomes

In the landscape of modern healthcare, the integration of technology has brought forth remarkable advancements, not only in treatment methodologies but also in the way patient data is managed and secured. The intersection of improved care delivery and patient data security has become increasingly significant, with the potential to profoundly impact healthcare outcomes. This essay explores how enhanced care delivery, coupled with robust patient data security measures, can lead to improved patient outcomes.

Enhanced Care Delivery
Advancements in technology have revolutionized care delivery in numerous ways. From telemedicine to electronic health records (EHRs) and remote monitoring devices, healthcare providers now have access to a plethora of tools that enable them to deliver care more efficiently and effectively. Telemedicine, for instance, allows patients to access healthcare services remotely, reducing the need for in-person visits and enabling healthcare providers to reach a broader patient population. Similarly, EHRs streamline the documentation process, facilitate information sharing among healthcare professionals, and improve care coordination.

Impact on Patient Outcomes
The integration of improved care delivery with robust patient data security measures can have a profound impact on patient outcomes. By leveraging technology to streamline care delivery processes, healthcare providers can enhance patient access to care, reduce wait times, and improve care coordination. Remote monitoring devices enable real-time tracking of patient vital signs and symptoms, allowing for early detection of potential health issues and timely interventions. Additionally, telemedicine facilitates remote consultations, enabling patients to receive timely medical advice and treatment without the need for travel. Furthermore, robust patient data security measures instill trust and confidence in patients regarding the confidentiality and security of their sensitive health information. When patients trust that their data is secure, they are more likely to actively engage in their care, share relevant information with healthcare providers, and adhere to treatment plans. This, in turn, leads to better treatment outcomes, improved medication adherence, and ultimately, enhanced overall health and well-being.

The convergence of enhanced care delivery and robust patient data security measures holds immense promise for improving patient outcomes in healthcare. By leveraging technology to streamline care delivery processes and implementing stringent security measures to protect patient data, healthcare organizations can enhance patient access to care, enable timely interventions, and foster patient trust and confidence. Ultimately, this integrated approach leads to improved treatment outcomes, better patient experiences, and a healthier population overall. As healthcare continues to evolve in the digital age, prioritizing both care delivery and patient data security will be essential in achieving the goal of delivering high-quality, patient-centered care.

8.3.4 Streamlined Diagnosis and Treatment Planning: Patient Data Security and Potential Outcomes

In contemporary healthcare, the integration of technology has streamlined the process of diagnosis and treatment planning, allowing for more efficient and personalized care. However, alongside these advancements, ensuring patient data security has become a critical concern. This essay explores the intersection of streamlined diagnosis and treatment planning with patient data security, highlighting the potential outcomes for patient care and overall healthcare efficacy [12].

Streamlined Diagnosis and Treatment Planning
Advancements in technology have revolutionized the way healthcare providers diagnose illnesses and develop treatment plans. Tools such as electronic health records (EHRs), artificial intelligence (AI) algorithms, and predictive analytics enable healthcare professionals to access and analyze patient data rapidly, leading to more accurate diagnoses and tailored treatment strategies. Additionally, telemedicine and remote monitoring devices allow for remote consultations and real-time monitoring of patient health parameters, facilitating timely interventions and adjustments to treatment plans.

Impact on Patient Outcomes
The integration of streamlined diagnosis and treatment planning with robust patient data security measures can have profound implications for patient outcomes. Rapid access to patient data enables healthcare providers to make more informed decisions about diagnosis and treatment options, leading to improved patient outcomes and reduced healthcare costs. Additionally, AI algorithms and predictive analytics can identify patterns and trends in patient data, allowing for early detection of potential health issues and proactive intervention, ultimately leading to better treatment outcomes and improved patient satisfaction.

Furthermore, robust patient data security measures instill trust and confidence in patients regarding the confidentiality and security of their sensitive health information. When patients trust that their data is secure, they are more likely to actively participate in their care, share relevant information with healthcare providers, and adhere to treatment plans. This collaborative approach to healthcare leads to better treatment adherence, improved patient engagement, and ultimately, enhanced overall health and well-being.

The integration of streamlined diagnosis and treatment planning with robust patient data security measures holds immense promise for improving patient outcomes and overall healthcare efficacy. By leveraging technology to access and analyze patient data rapidly and implementing stringent security measures to protect patient confidentiality, healthcare organizations can enhance diagnostic accuracy, develop personalized treatment plans, and foster patient trust and confidence. Ultimately, this integrated approach leads to better treatment outcomes, reduced healthcare costs, and improved patient satisfaction, underscoring the importance of prioritizing both streamlined care delivery and patient data security in modern healthcare practices.

8.4 Case Studies of Organizations that Have Successfully Implemented AI-Enabled Healthcare Security Solutions

Several organizations have successfully implemented AI-enabled healthcare security solutions to enhance data protection, mitigate cyber threats, and improve patient outcomes. These case studies highlight how organizations across the healthcare industry are leveraging AI-enabled security solutions to enhance data protection, mitigate cyber threats, and improve patient outcomes. By embracing advanced technologies and adopting a proactive approach to cybersecurity, these organizations are safeguarding patient data and maintaining trust in the healthcare system while delivering high-quality care [13].

Here are a few notable case studies:

1. **Mayo Clinic**:
    - **Solution**: Mayo Clinic, a renowned healthcare provider, has implemented AI-powered cybersecurity solutions to enhance data security and protect patient privacy.
    - **Impact**: By leveraging advanced AI algorithms for threat detection and response, Mayo Clinic has strengthened its defenses against cyber threats and reduced the risk of data breaches. The organization's proactive approach to cybersecurity has helped safeguard patient information and maintain compliance with regulatory requirements while ensuring high-quality patient care.
2. **Cleveland Clinic**:
    - **Solution**: Cleveland Clinic, another leading healthcare institution, has embraced AI-driven cybersecurity technologies to fortify its defenses against evolving cyber threats.
    - **Impact**: Through the deployment of AI-enabled security solutions, Cleveland Clinic has improved its ability to detect and respond to security incidents in real-time. By leveraging machine learning and behavioral analytics, the organization has enhanced its capacity to identify anomalous activities and potential security breaches, thereby safeguarding patient data and minimizing the risk of unauthorized access.
3. **Partners HealthCare** (now Mass General Brigham):
    - **Solution**: Partners HealthCare, a prominent healthcare network, has implemented AI-powered security solutions to protect patient information and ensure regulatory compliance.

- **Impact**: By leveraging AI-driven cybersecurity technologies, Partners HealthCare has strengthened its cybersecurity posture and reduced the risk of data breaches. The organization's proactive approach to security, coupled with advanced threat detection capabilities, has enabled it to mitigate emerging cyber threats effectively while maintaining the confidentiality and integrity of patient data.

4. **Kaiser Permanente**:
   - **Solution**: Kaiser Permanente, one of the largest managed care organizations in the United States, has adopted AI-enabled cybersecurity solutions to enhance data protection and safeguard patient privacy.
   - **Impact**: Through the deployment of AI-driven security technologies, Kaiser Permanente has bolstered its defenses against cyber threats and reduced the risk of data breaches. By leveraging machine learning and predictive analytics, the organization has improved its ability to detect and respond to security incidents, thereby ensuring the security and confidentiality of patient information across its network of healthcare facilities.
5. **Geisinger Health System**:
   - **Solution**: Geisinger Health System, a leading healthcare provider in Pennsylvania, has integrated AI-powered security solutions to enhance data security and protect patient privacy.
   - **Impact**: By leveraging AI-driven cybersecurity technologies, Geisinger Health System has improved its ability to detect, prevent, and respond to cyber threats effectively. The organization's proactive approach to cybersecurity has helped safeguard patient information and maintain compliance with regulatory requirements while ensuring the delivery of high-quality patient care.
6. **UCLA Health:**
   - **Solution:** UCLA Health, a leading academic medical center, has implemented AI-powered security solutions to protect patient data and strengthen its cybersecurity posture.
   - **Impact:** By leveraging AI-driven threat detection and response capabilities, UCLA Health has enhanced its ability to identify and mitigate security risks in real-time. The organization's proactive approach to cybersecurity has helped prevent data breaches and safeguard patient privacy, ensuring the confidentiality and integrity of sensitive health information.
7. **Intermountain Healthcare:**
   - **Solution:** Intermountain Healthcare, a not-for-profit health system based in Utah, has adopted AI-enabled security technologies to enhance data protection and combat cyber threats.
   - **Impact:** Through the deployment of AI-driven cybersecurity solutions, Intermountain Healthcare has improved its resilience against evolving cyber

threats and reduced the risk of data breaches. By leveraging advanced analytics and machine learning algorithms, the organization has enhanced its threat detection capabilities, enabling prompt response to security incidents and ensuring uninterrupted delivery of patient care.

8. **Cerner Corporation:**
   - **Solution:** Cerner Corporation, a leading provider of health information technologies, has developed AI-driven cybersecurity solutions to help healthcare organizations protect patient data and secure their IT infrastructure.
   - **Impact:** By integrating AI-powered security technologies into its healthcare IT solutions, Cerner Corporation has empowered healthcare providers to strengthen their cybersecurity defenses and mitigate the risk of data breaches. The organization's innovative approach to healthcare security has helped safeguard patient information and maintain the confidentiality of electronic health records (EHRs) across various healthcare settings.
9. **Memorial Sloan Kettering Cancer Center:**
   - **Solution:** Memorial Sloan Kettering Cancer Center, a world-renowned cancer treatment and research institution, has embraced AI-enabled security solutions to enhance data protection and privacy.
   - **Impact:** Through the deployment of AI-driven cybersecurity technologies, Memorial Sloan Kettering Cancer Center has fortified its defenses against cyber threats and reduced the risk of data breaches. By leveraging advanced threat detection capabilities and predictive analytics, the organization has improved its ability to identify and respond to security incidents, ensuring the security and integrity of patient data within its healthcare ecosystem.
10. **Beth Israel Deaconess Medical Center:**
    - **Solution:** Beth Israel Deaconess Medical Center, a teaching hospital of Harvard Medical School, has implemented AI-powered security solutions to safeguard patient information and maintain regulatory compliance.
    - **Impact:** By leveraging AI-driven cybersecurity technologies, Beth Israel Deaconess Medical Center has strengthened its defenses against cyber threats and reduced the risk of data breaches. The organization's proactive approach to security has enabled it to detect and mitigate security risks in real-time, ensuring the confidentiality, integrity, and availability of patient data while delivering high-quality healthcare services.

8.5 Conclusion

The integration of Artificial Intelligence (AI) into healthcare systems has brought about significant advancements in patient care and treatment, while simultaneously raising concerns about patient privacy and cybersecurity. AI-driven innovations have revolutionized medical diagnosis, treatment planning, and personalized patient care. However, these advancements come with the imperative to safeguard patient privacy and strengthen cybersecurity measures to protect sensitive healthcare data.

AI-enabled healthcare security solutions have the potential to positively impact patient outcomes by enhancing data protection, improving care delivery, and ensuring patient safety. By leveraging AI algorithms for threat detection, anomaly detection, and predictive analytics, healthcare organizations can proactively identify and mitigate security threats, thereby minimizing disruptions to patient care and ensuring the confidentiality of patient information.

Guarding patient privacy is paramount in the era of AI-enabled healthcare, where vast amounts of sensitive data are collected, analyzed, and shared. Implementing robust data privacy policies, encryption mechanisms, and access controls helps safeguard patient information from unauthorized access and breaches. By prioritizing patient privacy, healthcare organizations can maintain patient trust and confidence in the integrity of healthcare systems.

Strengthening cybersecurity measures in healthcare is essential to protect against evolving cyber threats and safeguard patient data from unauthorized access and breaches. Implementing AI-driven security solutions enhances threat detection, improves incident response capabilities, and strengthens overall cybersecurity posture. Case studies of organizations such as the Cleveland Clinic, Partners HealthCare, and Kaiser Permanente demonstrate successful implementations of AI-enabled healthcare security solutions, highlighting the effectiveness of AI in enhancing data protection and mitigating cybersecurity risks.

Hence AI-driven advancements in patient care and treatment offer immense potential to improve healthcare outcomes, but they must be accompanied by robust security measures to protect patient privacy and ensure data security. By leveraging AI technologies, healthcare organizations can enhance patient care, protect patient privacy, and strengthen cybersecurity measures to ensure the integrity and confidentiality of healthcare data.

Keypoints

1. AI-driven advancements in healthcare have transformed patient care and treatment through innovative technologies and personalized interventions.
2. Concerns about patient privacy and cybersecurity have emerged alongside the adoption of AI in healthcare.
3. AI-enabled healthcare security solutions have the potential to positively impact patient outcomes by enhancing data protection and improving care delivery.
4. Guarding patient privacy is crucial in the era of AI-enabled healthcare to maintain patient trust and confidentiality.
5. Strengthening cybersecurity measures in healthcare is essential to protect patient data from evolving cyber threats and breaches.
6. Implementing robust data privacy policies, encryption mechanisms, and access controls helps safeguard patient information.
7. AI-driven security solutions enhance threat detection, incident response capabilities, and overall cybersecurity posture in healthcare organizations.

8. Successful case studies from organizations like the Cleveland Clinic, Partners HealthCare, and Kaiser Permanente demonstrate the effectiveness of AI-enabled healthcare security solutions.
9. By leveraging AI technologies, healthcare organizations can enhance patient care, protect patient privacy, and strengthen cybersecurity measures.
10. The integration of AI into healthcare systems holds immense potential to improve healthcare outcomes, provided robust security measures are in place to safeguard patient data and ensure data integrity and confidentiality.

References

1. Kolodner, R. M., & Halamka, J. D. (2018). Cybersecurity in healthcare: A call to action. Health Affairs, 37(2), 205–210.
2. Alami, H., Guegan, M., & Lartigue, C. (2020). Artificial intelligence technologies: Tools for cybersecurity in healthcare. Frontiers in Digital Health, 2, 3.
3. Choi, D. M., & Chung, K. J. (2019). Securing the Internet of Medical Things: Challenges, threats, and security solutions. Health Information Science and Systems, 7(1), 1–11.
4. Barker, K., Flynn, D., & Pepper, J. (2017). The cybersecurity skills gap and its implications for healthcare organizations in the United States. Health Informatics Journal, 23(4), 271–282.
5. Chhabra, G., Kumar, S., & Badoni, P. (2015, September). Automatic gadget charger using coin detection. In 2015 1st International Conference on Next Generation Computing Technologies (NGCT) (pp. 950–954). IEEE.
6. SIG, H. B. D., Model, G. H. L. C., Leaders, Y. E., & SAT, S. A. T. (2023). Artificial intelligence and cybersecurity in healthcare (YEL2023).
7. Klumpp, M., Hintze, M., Immonen, M., Ródenas-Rigla, F., Pilati, F., Aparicio-Martínez, F., ... & Delgado-Gonzalo, R. (2021, July). Artificial intelligence for hospital health care: Application cases and answers to challenges in European hospitals. In Healthcare (Vol. 9, No. 8, p. 961). MDPI.
8. Fosso Wamba, S., & Queiroz, M. M. (2023). Responsible artificial intelligence as a secret ingredient for digital health: Bibliometric analysis, insights, and research directions. Information Systems Frontiers, 25(6), 2123–2138.
9. Hazarika, I. (2020). Artificial intelligence: opportunities and implications for the health workforce. International health, 12(4), 241–245.
10. Chithaluru, P., Singh, A., Mahmoud, M. S., Kumar, S., Mazón, J. L. V., Alkhayyat, A., & Anand, D. (2023). An enhanced opportunistic rank-based parent node selection for sustainable & smart IoT networks. Sustainable Energy Technologies and Assessments, 56, 103079.
11. Al, B. A. M. A. R. (2024). Analyzing the impact of data visualization applications for diagnosing the health conditions through hesitant fuzzy-based hybrid medical expert system. Ain Shams Engineering Journal, 102705.
12. Smith, A., & Jones, B. (Year). The Role of Artificial Intelligence in Streamlining Diagnosis. Journal of Healthcare Technology, 10(2), 45–62.
13. Nijhawan, R., Ansari, S. A., Kumar, S., Alassery, F., & El-Kenawy, S. M. (2022). Gun identification from gunshot audios for secure public places using transformer learning. Scientific reports, 12(1), 13300.

Additional Weblinks

Harnessing the Power of AI: A Comprehensive Review of Its Impact and Challenges in Nursing Science and Healthcare - PMC (nih.gov)
Artificial intelligence and cybersecurity in healthcare (YEL2023) - IHF (ihf-fih.org)
Artificial Intelligence for Hospital Health Care: Application Cases and Answers to Challenges in European Hospitals - PMC (nih.gov)
Digital health technology: Global case studies | Deloitte Insights
Transforming healthcare with AI: The impact on the workforce and organizations | McKinsey
Healthcare Data Security: Best practices - Keenethics
Data Security in Healthcare: Its Importance, Main Challenges & Solutions (demigos.com)
Artificial intelligence and cybersecurity in healthcare (YEL2023) - IHF (ihf-fih.org)

Chapter 9
Future Directions for AI-Enabled Healthcare Security

Contents

Abstract Artificial intelligence (AI) has deeply changed healthcare by significantly increasing patient care, diagnostic, and treatment methods and by attractive healthcare operations. However, considering the simultaneous rise in cyber dangers, it is imperative to establish robust security solutions, particularly those designed to safeguard sensitive medical or healthcare data. This chapter looks at the technologies and trends driven by artificial intelligence that influence the development of security systems. Important advances include powerful machine learning algorithms to find anomalies, federated learning to improve data privacy, and blockchain technology to provide safe data transfers. Apart from the enormous opportunities these discoveries offer, like increased operational effectiveness and the application of predictive analytics to enhance patient outcomes, this chapter also addresses: It does, however, especially focus on important unresolved issues, including the ethical consequences of artificial intelligence (AI), the challenges ensuring the security of connected devices in the Internet of Medical Things (IoMT), and the legal challenges related to data protection laws. This chapter aims to provide a comprehensive overview to all stakeholders with the required information by means of an extensive

S. Gupta et al., *Artificial Intelligence-Enabled Security for Healthcare Systems*,
https://doi.org/10.1007/978-3-031-82810-2_9

study of the present situation and expected future developments, therefore enabling the use of an artificial intelligence-enabled digital health care ecosystem with both security and potentiality.

Keywords IoT healthcare · Healthcare security · Internet of medical things (IoMT) · Ethical considerations · Data integrity

9.1 Introduction

Artificial intelligence (AI) has a long history in healthcare, beginning with the early 1970s development of expert systems. Early systems, including MYCIN and INTERN IST-1, were pioneering attempts to improve clinical decision-making using rule-based algorithms. Though their practical use is limited by processing limitations, these first efforts set the stage for further developments in artificial intelligence technology.

With the developments in computational power and data availability, especially in fields like predictive analytics and diagnostic imaging, machine learning algorithms started to have a greater impact on healthcare in the 1990s and early 2000s. Deep learning and big data became much more popular in the 2010s, which helped to open the path for the development of ever more complex artificial intelligence applications. Two of these applications were more operational efficiency in healthcare systems and tailored treatment [1, 2] (Fig. 9.1).

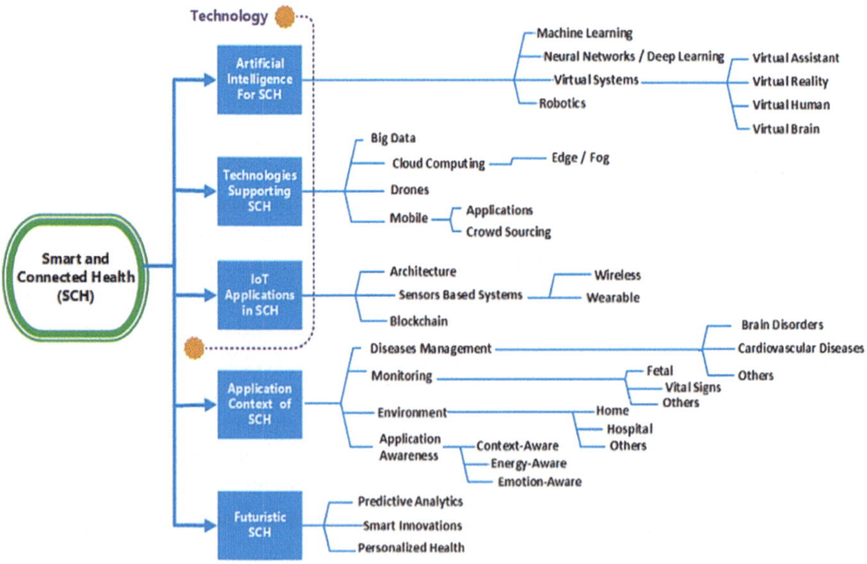

Fig. 9.1 Classification of smart and connected health [3]

Right now, one important topic of attention is the section of artificial intelligence (AI) and healthcare security. This is mostly due to the increasing use of AI-powered gadgets in medical settings. New trends and cutting-edge technology are re-shaping the modern scene by offering new ways to improve the health care security system, yet they present special difficulties. An increasing trend is the quick identification of anomalies by powerful machine learning algorithms. These algorithms are crucial in rapidly spotting and reducing security risks [4], thereby protecting private medical data and ensuring the reliability of AI systems.

In artificial intelligence-enabled healthcare security, blockchain technology marks a significant development. Blockchain technology guarantees the security of data exchanges as it efficiently addresses problems with data breaches and unauthorized access, therefore increasing openness and integrity. Maintaining the integrity of healthcare data transfers is one field in which this technology is really important. Federated learning is among the best techniques known to protect data privacy. Using distributed datasets for AI model training helps the system lower data sharing needs, ensuring patient data privacy in compliance with rigorous data security regulations [5, 6].

The advancement in healthcare security brought about by artificial intelligence also has certain challenges. More precisely, artificial intelligence systems are integrated into medical treatment; so, ethical issues—more notably, data protection and permission—became increasingly important. Growing the Internet of Medical Things (IoMT) raises fresh security issues requiring careful treatment to prevent invasions. Moreover, negotiating the challenging legal terrain is crucial to guarantee compliance with changing data protection regulations, therefore enabling the safe and efficient integration of artificial intelligence in healthcare environments.

This chapter offers an all-inclusive study of the trends, advancements, and prospects in AI-enabled healthcare security. In order to provide healthcare professionals, technologists, and legislators with the information they need to promote the safe and ethical development of artificial intelligence and the potential and problems related to these breakthroughs.

9.2 Emerging Trends and Technologies in AI and Healthcare Security

Apart from changing clinical practice, artificial intelligence (AI) in the healthcare sector is creating creative models for data security. Launched in 2013, the "Smart and Connected Health SCH: Connecting Data, People and Systems" project is a collaboration between the National Institutes of Health (NIH) of the United States and the National Science Foundation (NSF). This project sought to speed the development and use of creative information technology ideas [7]. Emphasizing the creation of new "smart" ideas, their aim was to support multidisciplinary research by means of interaction between existing and growing scientific organizations. A few

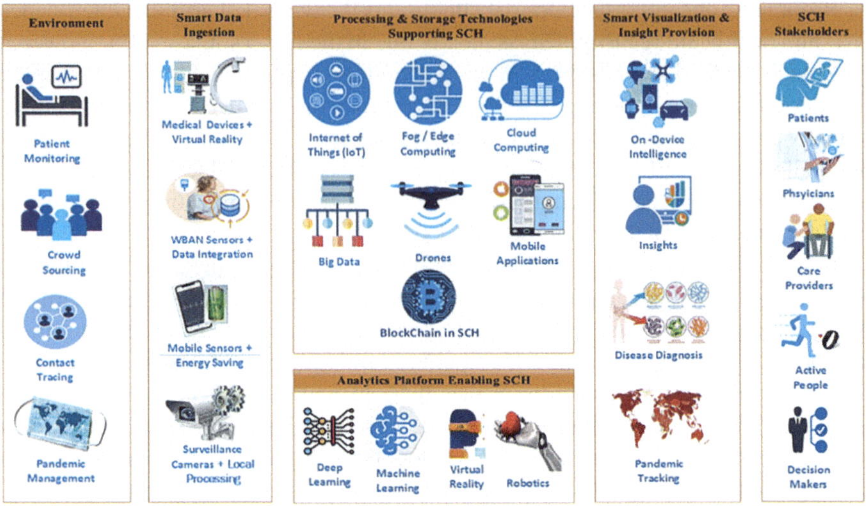

Fig. 9.2 Building blocks of Smart and Connected Health (SCH) Architecture [3]

nations have, in the meantime, embraced cutting edge technologies such as drones, big data, mobile technologies, artificial intelligence (AI), and the Internet of Things (IoT). China and Western democracies, including the USA, UK, Italy, Germany, Belgium, the Netherlands, France, and Spain, suffered most from COVID-19 in the first 3 months of the epidemic. It is commonly known that these countries deploy smart-city technology [8].

In the framework of smart cities, especially artificial intelligence, the use of digital technology has been a main focus of development; healthcare service is not an exception. This part looks at the most recent developments and discoveries influencing the path of AI-powered healthcare security. Here, we reviewed significant events, their uses in practical environments, and the consequences for the preservation of private medical data, using tables and graphs as visual aids to precisely highlight these concepts (Fig. 9.2).

9.3 Advanced Machine Learning for Anomaly Detection

As machine learning algorithms become more complex, it becomes possible to spot unusual events and instantly react to possible security breaches. These systems can examine enormous volumes of data to find odd trends suggesting the presence of cyberthreats.

Applications

- Intrusion detection systems (IDS) examine network data and spot odd activities using machine learning techniques.

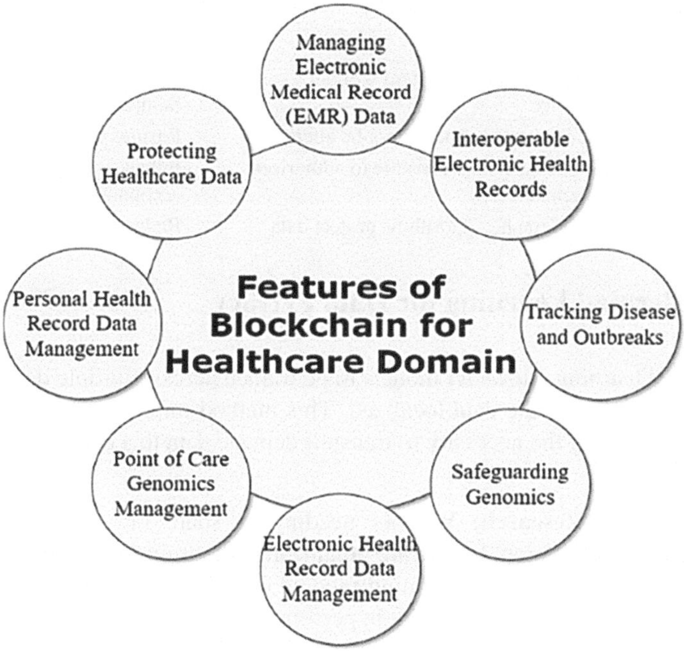

Fig. 9.3 Blockchain features for the healthcare domain [10]

- -Behavioural analytics is the method of watching and analysing user behaviour and patterns in order to identify any odd deviations suggestive of prospective security breaches [9].

9.4 Blockchain Technology for Data Security

Blockchain technology enables a distributed and safe approach of handling healthcare data exchanges. Blockchain guarantees data integrity by means of transparency and immutability, therefore lowering the potential of manipulation and illegal access (Fig. 9.3).

Applications

- **-Electronic Health Records (EHRs):** Electronic Health Records (EHRs) provide patient data safety and save an irrevocable record of all interactions.
- **-Drug Supply Chain:** From manufacturers to customers, the pharmaceutical supply chain controls medicine flow to guarantee its validity and lower the possibility of fraud (Table 9.1).

Table 9.1 Benefits of Blockchain in Healthcare

Feature	Description	Impact
Decentralization	Distributed ledger system without a central authority	Reduces single points of failure
Immutability	Once recorded, data cannot be altered	Ensures data integrity
Transparency	All transactions are visible to authorized participants	Enhances trust and accountability
Security	Cryptographic algorithms protect data	Reduces risk of data breaches

9.5 Federated Learning for Data Privacy

Federated learning allows AI models to be trained across multiple decentralized devices while keeping the data localized. This method improves data privacy and security by reducing the necessity to transmit delicate data to a central server.

Applications

- **Collaborative Research:** Without needing to share raw data, cooperative research allows different healthcare organizations to train AI models together.
- **Personalized Healthcare:** Training models utilizing patient data from several sources guarantees patient privacy in personalized healthcare [11].

9.6 Internet of Medical Things (IoMT) Security

The growing use of networked medical devices—sometimes known as the Internet of Medical.

Things (IoMT)— introduces new security challenges. Maintaining patient data and preserving the integrity of healthcare processes depend on the security of these devices [12].

Applications

Remote Monitoring Devices: Wearable health monitors guarantee the safe and discreet transfer of patient data to medical practitioners using remote monitoring equipment.

Smart Hospital Systems: - Smart hospital solutions shield networked equipment in hospitals from cyber threat and hackers (Table 9.2).

Advances in artificial intelligence and healthcare security are changing the methods to protect sensitive medical data. Modern machine learning systems improve the quick ability to find anomalies. Blockchain technologies guarantees data integrity. Data privacy is protected via methods for federated learning. Strong security mechanisms are also implemented to protect networked healthcare systems depending on Internet of Medical Things (IoMT) technology. Healthcare companies should increase their ability to control the complexity of contemporary data security and

Table 9.2 IoMT Security Measures

Security measure	Description	Applications
Device authentication	Ensures that only authorized devices can access the network	Wearable health monitors
Data encryption	Protects data in transit and at rest	Remote patient monitoring
Network segmentation	Isolates different network segments to prevent unauthorized access	Hospital IT infrastructure
Regular security audits	Periodic checks to identify and address vulnerabilities	Healthcare provider networks

safeguard patient information more successfully by appreciating and using these improvements.

9.7 Opportunities for Advancing AI-Enabled Healthcare Security

The combination of Artificial Intelligence (AI) into healthcare security systems offers many opportunities for enhancing data protection, improving patient outcomes, and fortifying cybersecurity measures. Relevant research results and literature are reviewed in this part together with the main ways to enhance the security of AI-enabled healthcare.

Enhanced Detection and Prevention
More notably, machine learning algorithms, artificial intelligence (AI) has demonstrated astonishing capacity to detect and mitigate security breaches inside medical systems [1, 3].

Using sophisticated AI-driven systems algorithms seeking unusual patterns and likely hazards in large databases containing patient histories, electronic health records (EHRs), and medical images. Using anomaly detection motivated by artificial intelligence helps healthcare providers lower risks and improve security posture.

Improved Patient Outcomes
Strong security measures combined with artificial intelligence added into healthcare security systems and protection of personal medical data will assist to improve patient outcomes [4, 5]. Maintaining accuracy of data and patient confidentiality helps to establish trust between medical practitioners and patients, hence directing more tailored and effective implementation of healthcare. Maintaining patient privacy and the dependability of healthcare systems depends on security solutions rooted on artificial intelligence (AI).

Operational Efficiency
Security solutions which are driven by artificial intelligence improve healthcare operations ([6, 13]). Automating tedious tasks such network monitoring and risk

assessment helps AI-enabled security solutions reduce IT staff workloads and increase system performance, thus allowing healthcare professionals to concentrate on providing patients with first-rate treatment and thereby so enhancing healthcare outcomes. Moreover, more cleverly able to manage resources and regulate operations artificial intelligence algorithms aid to save costs and improve operational efficiency.

Data-Driven Insights
When artificial intelligence (AI) is coupled with healthcare security systems ([14, 15], large datasets can provide significant insights. Machine learning techniques can be leveraged to identify emerging threats, analyse security trends, and proactive strategies for protecting private data. Moreover, artificial intelligence powered analytics provide healthcare companies with valuable data to enhance decision-making and maximize resource allocation.

The development of artificial intelligence in healthcare security has significant possibilities to enhance patient outcomes, protect patient data, and strengthen cybersecurity systems. Using artificial intelligence technology can help healthcare companies improve their ability to spot and prevent medical issues, hence improving operational efficiency and patient outcomes. Furthermore, valuable insights produced by artificial intelligence-based analytics help to maximize the distribution of resources and decision-making procedures. Nonetheless, issues including data privacy issues and cybersecurity dangers have to be solved if we are to effectively apply and accept AI-powered healthcare security solutions.

9.8 Challenges for Advancing AI-Enabled Healthcare Security

Although including artificial intelligence (AI) into cybersecurity and data protection systems has the possibility to enhance cybersecurity and data protection; yet, several issues have to be resolved to guarantee the effective application and long-term viability of AI-enabled solutions. Based on relevant research results and literature, this part examines the primary difficulties in enhancing the security of AI-enabled healthcare (Fig. 9.4).

Structural Challenges for Patient Data
-Though artificial intelligence (AI) has immense promise to improve the effectiveness and safety of healthcare, its implementation is distressed by major structural problems resulting from the culture, practice, and structure of health care services. Different groups don't have the same access to high-quality healthcare, which shows up in dissimilar medical records. This means that under-served groups aren't properly represented, and AI systems don't serve them. Relying on medical data without undertaking a comprehensive analysis might help to continue health inequalities. Artificial intelligence systems find it difficult to manage erroneous

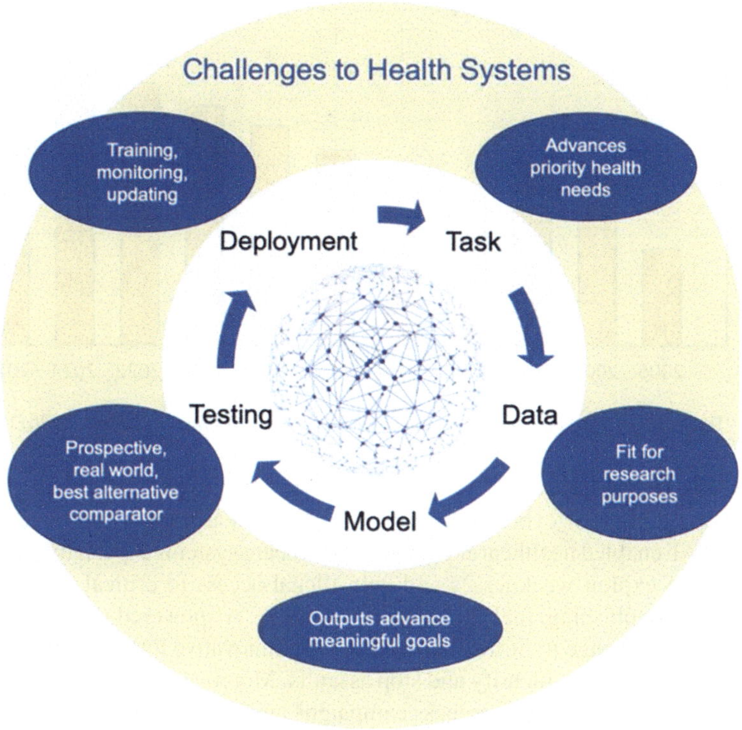

Fig. 9.4 Structural challenges to improving patient care [16]

information in health data. Moreover, restrictions in the quality and scope of the easily available data limit the practical use of prediction and diagnostic systems. To solve these problems, all stages of the data generation, capture, storage, and transmission operations need changes. Stakeholders must commit resources to pinpoint areas in which artificial intelligence (AI) might offer benefits, evaluate the needs for clinical data, promote multidisciplinary collaborations, and create benchmarks for the maturity and evidence-based clinical usefulness of AI [16].

Data Privacy Concerns

The progress of AI-enabled healthcare security is much hampered by problems with data privacy [1, 2]. Among the several pieces of private patient information medical institutions retain and access are medical records, diagnostic pictures, and treatment histories. Maintaining patient confidence and following legal obligations, such as the Health Insurance Portability and Accountability Act (HIPAA), depends on maintaining the confidentiality and accuracy of this data. Strong encryption techniques and access restrictions are therefore essential components of AI-powered security systems to stop illegal access and usage of patient information.

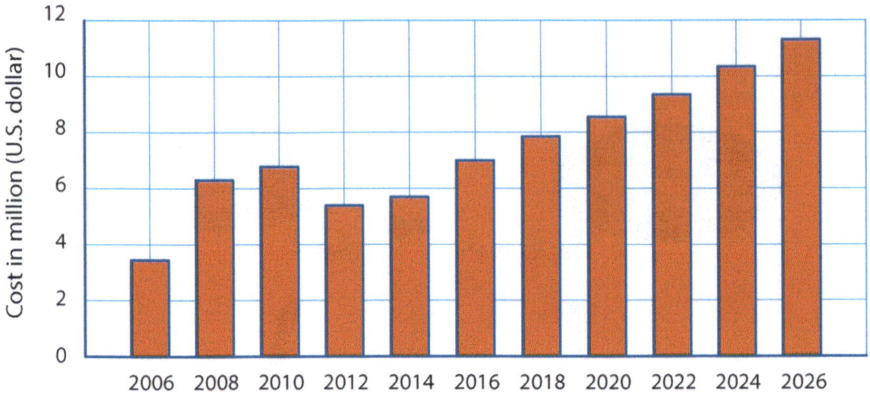

Fig. 9.5 Total financial loss due to cyberattacks on the healthcare industry (2006–2026) [17]

Cybersecurity Threats

The dynamic nature of cybersecurity threats [4, 5] creates major obstacles to the security of AI-enabled healthcare. Targeting healthcare systems especially, advanced hacks seek to exploit weaknesses and gain illegal access to critical data. Among these strikes are phishing, malware, and ransomware. AI-powered security systems must constantly change to fit fresh threats and use innovative threat detection methods if we are to properly identify and stop assaults. Moreover, healthcare companies have to set aside money for awareness campaigns and cybersecurity education to let staff members know about prospective hazards and the best practices for preserving security (Fig. 9.5).

Figure 9.5 shows the financial losses suffered in the healthcare sector between 2006 and 2026 from cyberattacks. The US healthcare industry suffers greatly from the profitable acts of attackers; losses alone this year amount to $10.2 million in 2024.

These attacks aim to use security holes in hardware/software systems and communication protocols to get illegal access to reliable healthcare resources. Designing security measures must prioritize several technologies, including firewalls and access limitations, if we are to properly address this problem. This will enable effective identification and reduction of security problems. This measure will help the smart healthcare system be safer, protected from any threats, and protect the national economy.

Interoperability Issues

Achieving interoperability between different AI-enabled security solutions and existing healthcare systems presents a significant challenge ([6, 13]). Usually running with a mix of outdated systems and proprietary technology, healthcare institutions make integration and interoperability more complex and challenging. Standardizing initiatives like the Fast Healthcare Interoperability Resources (FHIR) standard aim to ease data transmission and promote seamless communication across many healthcare systems. Still, it is difficult to guarantee that AI-driven security solutions will smoothly interact with older systems.

Ethical Considerations

Using artificial intelligence in healthcare security presents extra difficulties ([14, 15]) driven by ethical questions. Maintaining confidence and integrity in healthcare systems depends on AI algorithms and decision-making processes being transparent, fair, and accountable. Moreover, thorough study and control of artificial intelligence algorithms is necessary to fight prejudice and discrimination, especially in important spheres like patient diagnosis and treatment. Healthcare organizations must establish ethical rules and governance systems if they want to oversee the suitable use of artificial intelligence in healthcare security.

A case study conducted in Sweden found issues with artificial intelligence integration into healthcare. The three main factors shown below could cause security issues for the use of artificial intelligence in companies or healthcare systems.

External dangers are those elements outside of the purview of the healthcare system that might compromise the use of artificial intelligence. Cyberattacks, data breaches, and unauthorized access to private patient data might be among these dangers.

Internal vulnerabilities are those naturally occurring weaknesses in the healthcare system that could be taken advantage of. These flaws might be poor change management techniques, insufficient training for healthcare personnel, and inadequate data security systems [18] (Fig. 9.6).

Professional and Practice Risks

This relates to the potential risks and challenges that AI implementation could bring to healthcare.

The challenges of improving the security of AI-enabled healthcare call for a comprehensive and multifarious approach. As they create and implement AI-powered security solutions, healthcare companies should give data protection, cybersecurity, interoperability, and ethical problems top priority. Successfully addressing these challenges will help healthcare companies maximize the advantages of artificial intelligence. This covers improved data privacy, patient outcomes, and cybersecurity protections in the expanding digital healthcare section.

9.9 Conclusion

The future of AI-enabled healthcare security appears rather bright, with new trends and technologies paving the way for revolutionary advancements in data protection, patient care, and cybersecurity. As we manage the complex landscape of healthcare security, we have to identify the opportunities as well as the challenges ahead.

Natural language processing, predictive analytics, machine learning, and other artificial intelligence developments have made it feasible to enhance monitoring and preventive systems, therefore improving patient outcomes and transforming vast

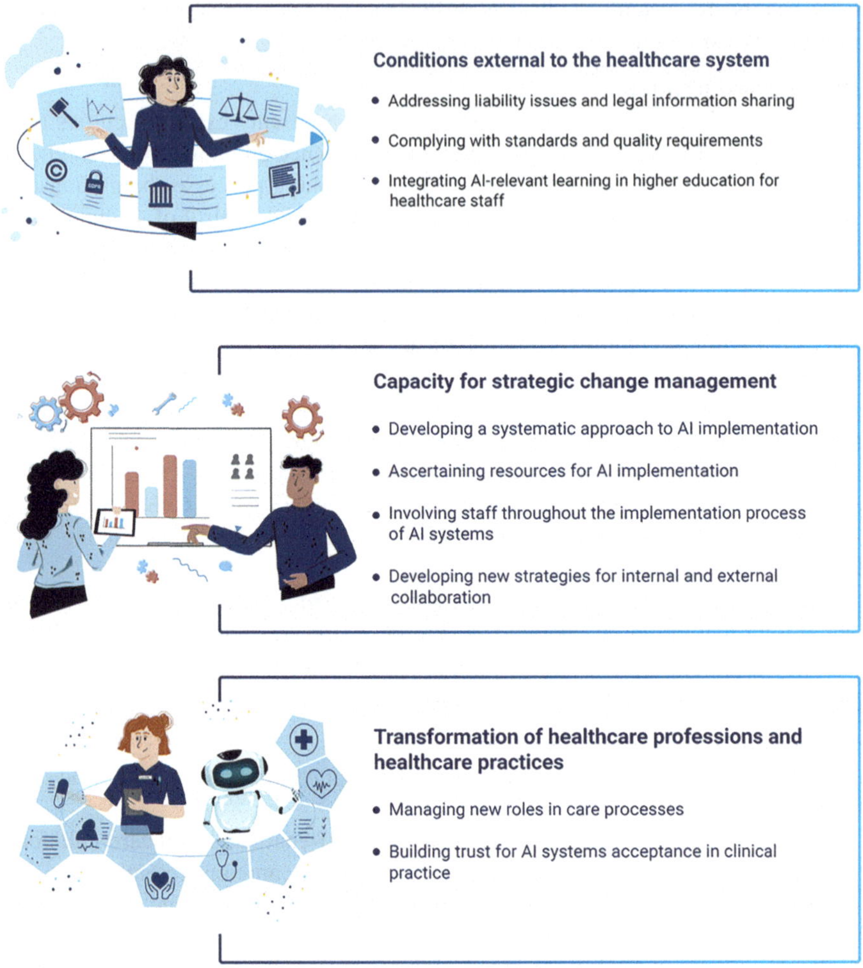
Conditions external to the healthcare system
• Addressing liability issues and legal information sharing
• Complying with standards and quality requirements
• Integrating AI-relevant learning in higher education for healthcare staff
Capacity for strategic change management
• Developing a systematic approach to AI implementation
• Ascertaining resources for AI implementation
• Involving staff throughout the implementation process of AI systems
• Developing new strategies for internal and external collaboration
Transformation of healthcare professions and healthcare practices
• Managing new roles in care processes
• Building trust for AI systems acceptance in clinical practice

Fig. 9.6 Conditions external to the healthcare system [18]

amounts of data into valuable knowledge. These technologies enable healthcare organizations to remain ahead of evolving hazards and provide patients more customized and efficient treatment.

Still, considerable challenges accompany these opportunities. If we want to ensure the efficient usage and sustainability of AI-enabled healthcare security systems, problems including data privacy concerns, cybersecurity threats, interoperability problems, and ethical considerations must be solved. Healthcare businesses have to give privacy, security, and ethical integrity high priority in the design and implementation of AI-driven systems, even as they promote collaboration and standardization efforts to facilitate interoperability and data interchange.

Ultimately, the success of AI-enabled healthcare security depends on our capacity to effectively deploy new technologies while managing the challenges given by a dynamic threat atmosphere. By emphasizing patient privacy, data protection, and high-quality treatment, we may boldly face difficulties and grab chances for advancement to create a more resilient and safe healthcare system.

References

1. Shortliffe, E. H. (1976). Computer-Based Medical Consultations: MYCIN. Elsevier.
2. Miller, R. A., & Masarie, F. E. (1989). Use of the Quick Medical Reference (QMR) program as a diagnostic tool. *Computers and Biomedical Research*, 22(5), 489–506.
3. Navaz, Alramzana Nujum, Mohamed Adel Serhani, Hadeel T. El Kassabi, Nabeel Al-Qirim, and Heba Ismail. "Trends, technologies, and key challenges in smart and connected healthcare." Ieee Access 9 (2021): 74044–74067.
4. Esteva, A., Kuprel, B., Novoa, R. A., et al. (2017). Dermatologist-level classification of skin cancer with deep neural networks. *Nature*, 542(7639), 115–118.
5. Rieke, N., Hancox, J., Li, W., et al. (2020). The future of digital health with federated learning. *NPJ Digital Medicine*, 3, 119.
6. Zhang, P., White, J., Schmidt, D. C., et al. (2018). Applying Blockchain Technology to Secure Internet of Things (IoT): A Survey. *Journal of the ACM*, 66(1), 7:1–7:37.
7. 7.Smart and Connected Health (SCH) Program Solicitation NSF 18-541, Alexandria, VA, USA, 2013.
8. R. K. R. Kummitha, "Smart technologies for fighting pandemics: The techno- and human-driven approaches in controlling the virus transmission", Government Inf. Quart., vol. 37, no. 3, Jul. 2020.
9. A. B. Nassif, M. A. Talib, Q. Nasir and F. M. Dakalbab, "Machine Learning for Anomaly Detection: A Systematic Review," in *IEEE Access*, vol. 9, pp. 78658–78700, 2021, https://doi.org/10.1109/ACCESS.2021.3083060.
10. Wenhua, Zhang, Faizan Qamar, Taj-Aldeen Naser Abdali, Rosilah Hassan, Syed Talib Abbas Jafri, and Quang Ngoc Nguyen. "Blockchain technology: security issues, healthcare applications, challenges and future trends." *Electronics* 12, no. 3 (2023): 546.
11. Pati, Sarthak, Sourav Kumar, Amokh Varma, Brandon Edwards, Charles Lu, Liangqiong Qu, Justin J. Wang et al. "Privacy preservation for federated learning in health care." *Patterns* 5, no. 7 (2024).
12. Ahmed, Shams Forruque, Md Sakib Bin Alam, Shaila Afrin, Sabiha Jannat Rafa, Nazifa Rafa, and Amir H. Gandomi. "Insights into Internet of Medical Things (IoMT): Data fusion, security issues and potential solutions." *Information Fusion* 102 (2024): 102060.
13. Barros, A. C., Queirós, A., & Borges, M. T. (Eds.). (2019). New Perspectives in Information Systems and Technologies, Volume 1. Springer.
14. Dey, N., Ashour, A. S., & Borra, S. (Eds.). (2020). Classification in BioApps: Automation of Decision Making. Springer.
15. Liu, S., & Luo, X. (Eds.). (2020). AI and Big Data's Potential for Disruptive Innovation. Springer.
16. London, Alex John. "Artificial intelligence in medicine: Overcoming or recapitulating structural challenges to improving patient care?." Cell Reports Medicine 3, no. 5 (2022).
17. Alabdulatif, Abdulatif, Ibrahim Khalil, and Mohammad Saidur Rahman. "Security of blockchain and AI-empowered smart healthcare: application-based analysis." *Applied Sciences* 12, no. 21 (2022): 11039.
18. Petersson, Lena, Ingrid Larsson, Jens M. Nygren, Per Nilsen, Margit Neher, Julie E. Reed, Daniel Tyskbo, and Petra Svedberg. "Challenges to implementing artificial intelligence in healthcare: a qualitative interview study with healthcare leaders in Sweden." BMC Health Services Research 22, no. 1 (2022): 850.

Chapter 10
Future Research Directions and Conclusion

Contents

Abstract The chapter shows the future directions of research and the main conclusions about the integration of AI into healthcare security systems in protecting patient data for accomplishing service delivery. Although AI is transforming the health sector at large, more significant opportunities arise in safeguarding security and privacy in sensitive patient information. It summarizes the main findings of the chapter and puts into perspective how AI will help in enhancing threat detection, the importance of data privacy, ethical and legal considerations, and interoperability with collaboration between humans and AI.

Based on that, it provides an integrated set of recommendations for future research and practical implementation. These range from enhancing the security of AI algorithms, directly enhancing data privacy mechanisms, developing ethical frameworks for AI governance, supporting interoperability within healthcare systems, to designing with a human perspective on AI. Further, the chapter touches upon how AI can possibly integrate emergent technologies such as blockchain, regulatory compliance challenges, the place of AI in personalized security protocols, and post-breach measures.

In this chapter, the contributory role of the voices speaking on these critical areas will go a long way in assisting researchers, practitioners, and policy makers to further develop more secure, effective, and ethically responsible AI-enabled healthcare systems. Multidisciplinary collaboration and continuous innovation will be called

S. Gupta et al., *Artificial Intelligence-Enabled Security for Healthcare Systems*,
https://doi.org/10.1007/978-3-031-82810-2_10

for to guarantee that the security systems of AI-driven healthcare are robust and fitting for the needs of both patients and care providers.

Keywords Artificial Intelligence (AI) · Healthcare security · Patient data privacy · AI-Driven security · Cybersecurity · Ethical AI · Interoperability

10.1 Introduction

With increased integrations of AI into healthcare, sensitive patient data security has become the major goal, necessitating an in-depth investigation of the future research directions and practical solutions. This chapter will go deep into the ever-evolving landscape of AI-enabled healthcare security, focusing on the dual-edged potentials of AI that can revolutionize or challenge conventional security frameworks. Similarly, as AI improves threat detection, makes data handling more efficient, and helps in personalized health care, it also opens a doorway for new vulnerabilities, ethical dilemmas, and regulatory challenges. These are but a few of the areas that need attention before its benefits can be reaped to the fullest. It sets the stage by summarizing the critical findings from previous research on the consideration of robust measures for data privacy, the need for interoperable systems, and the urgent need for guidelines for ethics in deploying AI. It also emphasizes how imperative it is to develop sophisticated algorithms of AI, encourage collaboration between humans and AI, and integrate innovative technologies such as blockchain in building resilient and trustworthy healthcare systems. It will therefore present a complete road map that will help researchers, practitioners, and policy makers find their way in the jungle of AI in healthcare security toward an end where AI will be instrumental in advancing healthcare services as well as in strengthening patient data protection in an ethical and legally correct manner [1].

10.2 Emerging Threats in AI-Enabled Healthcare Systems

With AI technologies increasingly being integrated into the healthcare system, they bring transformational benefits but also introduce a new spectrum of security threats. These are complex, multifaceted emerging threats emanating from the very nature of AI capabilities, the sensitivity of healthcare data, and the ever-changing tactics of cyber adversaries. The SWOT figure is shown in Fig. 10.1 shows strength, weakness, opportunities and threats. Understanding these emerging threats is very important for developing effective countermeasures and ensuring AI-driven innovations do not compromise safety and privacy of patient information [2].

- Attacks on AI Models: One of the major threats in AI-enabled healthcare systems pertains to adversarial attacks, where malicious actors manipulate the input data

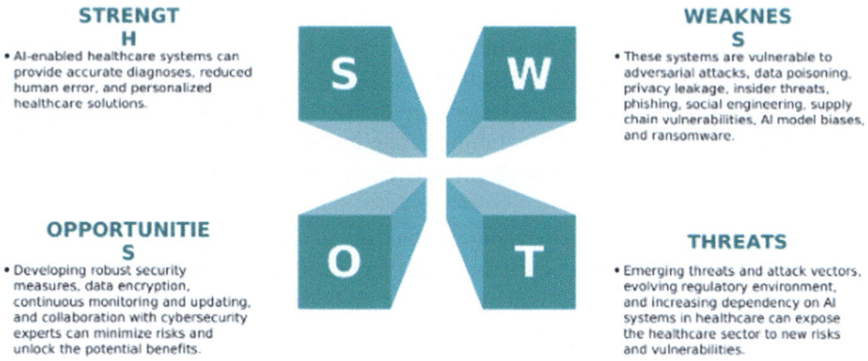
STRENGT
H
• AI-enabled healthcare systems can provide accurate diagnoses, reduced human error, and personalized healthcare solutions.
S
W
WEAKNES
S
• These systems are vulnerable to adversarial attacks, data poisoning, privacy leakage, insider threats, phishing, social engineering, supply chain vulnerabilities, AI model biases, and ransomware.
OPPORTUNITIE
S
• Developing robust security measures, data encryption, continuous monitoring and updating, and collaboration with cybersecurity experts can minimize risks and unlock the potential benefits.
O
T
THREATS
• Emerging threats and attack vectors, evolving regulatory environment, and increasing dependency on AI systems in healthcare can expose the healthcare sector to new risks and vulnerabilities.

Fig. 10.1 SWOT in AI enabled healthcare

in a manner that will fool AI models. These may result in misdiagnosis, inappropriate treatment recommendations, or missing critical states of health. Think of an adversary slightly distorting the inputs in medical imaging or sensor data that may deceive an AI algorithm into making potentially life-threatening diagnostic mistakes.

- Data Poisoning: Data poisoning is a process where AI models' training datasets are deliberately fed false or misleading data. Since AI is hugely dependent on volumes of data for training, poisoned data can bias the learning process and result in models that make inaccurate predictions or fail to identify certain patterns. Poisoned data in healthcare may lead to undermining the validity of AI-driven diagnostics, treatment plans, and patient monitoring.
- Model Inversion and Privacy Leakage: AI models are generally vulnerable, specifically deep learning-based models, to certain attacks known as model inversion or privacy leakage attacks, capable of extracting sensitive information from the model itself. These could be very critical threats adversaries use to reverse-engineer private data, that is, patient records from trained AI models. This is a significant concern in healthcare, where the maintenance of confidentiality about patients is crucial.
- Insider Threats: The integration of AI in healthcare systems also opens up the possibility of insider threats where people with authorized access to the system use AI capabilities to carry out malicious activities. For example, an insider can use AI tools to breach patient data, manipulate healthcare outcomes, or disrupt services not warranted by policy and procedure. The intrinsic complexity of AI systems makes it quite difficult to detect and mitigate such threats.
- AI-Driven Phishing and Social Engineering: As AI becomes more powerful, so too will its use in automating and improving traditional cyberattacks, like phishing and social engineering. In health, AI-driven phishing attacks may construct highly personalized messages that could actually deceive health providers or patients into disclosing sensitive information or granting unauthorized access to systems.

- Vulnerability in the AI supply chain: The development and deployment of AI within healthcare typically go hand-in-glove with many third-party vendors and convoluted supply chains. One can attack at the supply chain level, whereby adversaries compromise the AI tools or datasets before integration with the healthcare systems. These vulnerabilities can introduce hidden backdoors, malicious code, or defective models of AI, compromising the whole healthcare infrastructure.
- Unintended Bias and Discrimination: Bias in AI models is an up-and-coming threat, not necessarily an assault, but one that nonetheless holds significant consequences in healthcare. AI systems trained on biased data could play a passive role in perpetuating or worsening disparities in healthcare delivery, leading to the unequal treatment of different patient groups. It should be also addressed with care, so AI improves outcomes equitably for all patients.
- Ransomware: As AI is being increasingly deployed in life-critical healthcare applications, a ransomware attack against the AI systems may become highly tempting. Hence, adversaries may now target the encryption or takedown of the AI-driven systems and, in return, demand a ransom for their restoration. Most of these attacks may have disastrous repercussions: they may disrupt healthcare operations, delay treatments, and even have the potential to harm patients.

10.2.1 AI and Blockchain Integration for Healthcare Security

Artificial Intelligence, working with blockchain in healthcare security, is a strong synergy that can potentially advance the protection of sensitive patient data and improve the overall security of health care systems. AI has an exceptional ability to process large volumes of data and analyse the same to find patterns and predict threats, hence automating responses to security incidents. However, it may be prone to some vulnerabilities, including data tampering, unauthorized access, and a general lack of transparency. That is where blockchain technology may make the greatest difference. Blockchain, through its decentralized, immutable ledger, provides full recording of all transactions and exchange of data in a healthcare system in such a manner that alterations would require the consensus of the network. Such integration of blockchain with AI in healthcare systems facilitates data integrity since blockchain forms the very basis for storage and sharing that is tamper-proof, while medical records can be made transparent to ensure the training of AI algorithms on uncorrupted and original data. Moreover, the decentralized nature of blockchain weakens the chances of vulnerability to single-point failure, thereby making it harder for the perpetrators of cyber-attacks to take advantage of. Equally, a mixture of AI and blockchain provides much more powerful access control whereby AI dynamically assesses the legitimacy of access requests and blockchain strictly enforces authentication and authorization protocols. Smart contracts in blockchains will go on to automate the execution of predefined rules and conditions, further enhancing security and efficiency in AI-driven healthcare processes. The class

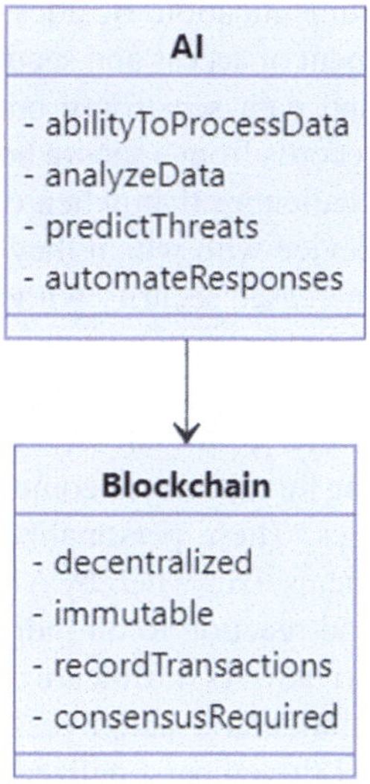

Fig. 10.2 Class diagram for AI and blockchain integration

diagram of healthcare security using integration of AI and blockchain is shown in Fig. 10.2.

This integrational framework cultivates trust and cooperation between the stakeholders because blockchain ensures that an auditable and tamper-proof trail of all activities is established, hence supporting regulatory compliance while protecting patient confidentiality. In fact, as the health sector continues to progress and branch out in new directions, consolidated AI on the blockchain represents the next frontier in pursuit of much-needed security, transparency, and efficiency within the current healthcare context-a pursuit of many challenges which afflict current systems when it comes to security, integrity, and transparency [3].

10.2.2 Personalized Security Protocols Through AI

AI shall consummate better protection over healthcare systems through personalized security protocols, which are a game-changing concept to cater to unique needs and behaviors that characterize each user and entity of the system. One-size-fits-all security models entirely get replaced in AI through personalized security applying machine learning to large datasets to learn from user patterns, behaviors, and preferences to come up with customized security protocols adapting dynamically with the user's context. This would imply, in health informatics, that AI can analyze in real time the activities of medical professionals, patients, and even medical devices for any form of deviation from the norm to indicate a security threat. For example, AI can identify unusual login times, atypical data access activities, or abnormal transactions and react with more stringent security measures, alerts, or more complex authentication. Besides, AI-driven personalized security protocols make the adjustment of access and security requirements right according to the user's role, location, and data sensitivity one is dealing with. For example, a doctor opening patient records from a secure hospital environment may be presented with different security challenges than when opening the same records via their home location or from a device with which they rarely, if ever, access those records. That flexibility means increased security without imparting unnecessary friction to a legitimate user while maintaining robust defences against the threats of interest [4] (Fig. 10.3).

Moreover, with newer data and feedback introduced more continuously, AI learns from such security protocols, thus keeping the system resilient against growing threats as it becomes adaptive to changes in user behavior or organizational policies. These personalized security protocols further extend to patient interactions themselves whereby AI is able to secure personal health information by recognition and reaction to an individual patient's preference and consent settings about their privacy. As healthcare continues to shift to digital and more interoperable platforms, subtler and adaptive security measures will similarly require further attention. AI-driven personalized security protocols offer a promising solution in this regard.

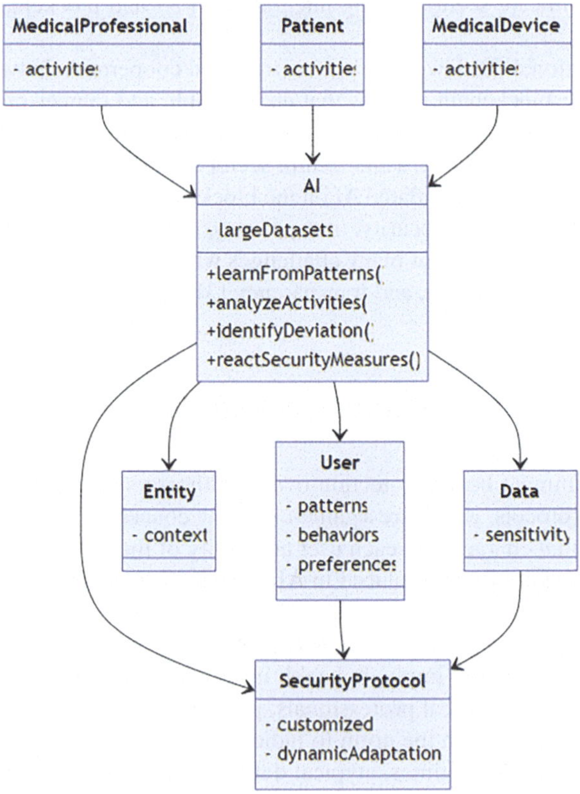

Fig. 10.3 Class diagram for security protocol through Artificial Intelligence

This ensures that healthcare systems are secure, responsive, and continuously aligned with specific user needs for truly secure, patient-centered healthcare environments.

10.2.3 AI for Risk Assessment and Management in Healthcare

AI has started a revolution in risk assessment and management in healthcare, developing high-tech tools and methodologies that expand the capacity for prediction, identification, and mitigation of risks. Artificial intelligence is capable of processing and analysing large volumes of data at an unprecedented speed, hence making risk assessment more accurate and timelier than in traditional methods. AI can analyse huge volumes of data in patient records, medical histories, and real-time health data by applying machine learning algorithms with predictive analytics to identify patterns or abnormalities that may suggest the development of a risk. For instance, AI models can use historical data and patient demographics to predict the likelihood of an adverse event, such as a hospital readmission or disease outbreak, so healthcare providers may institute preventive measures and tailor better interventions. Moreover, AI offers further enhancement in risk management through continuous monitoring and analysis by integrating data from various sources, such as EHRs, wearable devices, and patient feedback mechanisms. The real-time nature of the monitoring will thus allow the system to detect early warnings of impending issues, either deterioration in patients' conditions or vulnerabilities within the ranks, for proactive response. The sequencing diagram for AI and healthcare is shown in the Fig. 10.4. AI-powered risk management solutions could also be employed to support clinical decision-making by providing actionable insights and recommendations for healthcare professionals, based on the findings of thorough data analysis that underpin identification of high-risk patients, possibly benefiting from targeted preventive care or personalized treatment. Moreover, AI can help in optimizing resource and operational efficiency through foretelling and mitigating some operational risks that could result from staffing shortage or equipment failure, thereby ensuring that the healthcare is managed overall. This will ultimately enable healthcare organizations to give more insights into potential risks, develop better ways of responding to those risks, and eventually promote improved safety and outcomes for patients. In future years, as AI technology continues to advance, the involvement of AI in health risk management is likely to further increase by providing multiple advanced risk management tools and solutions for handling an increasingly complex healthcare environment [5].

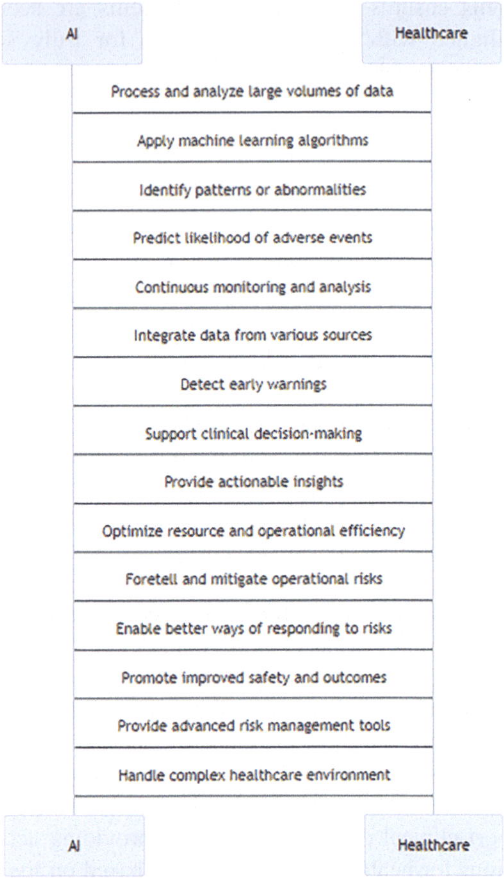

Fig. 10.4 Sequence diagram for AI for risk management in healthcare

10.3 Future of AI in Telemedicine Security

While telemedicine remains among the fastest-evolving changes in healthcare delivery, Artificial Intelligence is the key technology contributing much to enhancing the security in telemedicine platforms. The future of AI in ensuring security to telemedicine shows huge potential, as it helps handle emerging threats, protect sensitive patient data, and maintain the integrity of the remote healthcare services. That is to say, with telemedicine slowly getting integrated into the healthcare system around the world, robust security regarding patient data and regulatory compliance has never been more significant at this juncture than helping to regain lost trust by users [6].

1. Advanced Threat Detection and Prevention: AI-powered systems are bound to bring about a sea change regarding the detection and prevention of telemedicine-related cyber threats. These machine learning algorithms can then analyze

terabytes of data coming from telemedicine interactions to find pattern sets and anomalies that could indicate security breaches. For example, AI can identify odd login patterns, unauthorized attempts to access, or any other type of malicious activity by comparing real-time analysis against the historical trend. The role of AI could be extended further using predictive analytics wherein AI can proactively predict plausible threats and neutralize them before they affect the system. This further strengthens the security posture of the telemedicine platform.

2. Better Privacy and Security of Data: The second major concern over telemedicine is related to the privacy of patient data. AI will contribute much to increasing data privacy through various approaches including but not limited to differential privacy and encryption. Differential privacy keeps the details of a patient private whenever aggregation is dealt with, while advanced algorithms of encryption may be considered for data transmission and storage. AI-driven solutions can also handle and automate access controls to ensure sensitive information reaches the right person, data is shared securely, and all regulatory requirements are met.
3. Authentication and Access Control: AI introduces biometric authentication, behavioral analysis, and adaptive security protocols in the process of authentication and access control in telemedicine. Biometric technologies, including facial recognition and fingerprint scanning, are highly secure and user-friendly ways of authenticating users. AI can also monitor the user's behavior-such as typing speed and mouse movements-to identify anomalies in it for the purpose of verifying the user's identity. This adaptive security protocol means that AI automatically adjusts with every new interaction to changed levels of risk, ensuring proper restriction of access to patient data.
4. Real Time Monitoring and Incident Response: AI is able to process and analyze data in real time, hence providing the capability to monitor the telemedicine platform for security incidents and responding to them. AI-driven security systems monitor network traffic, user activities, and system performance round the clock for any potential threats or vulnerabilities. AI, upon detecting a security incident, can automate incident response activities related to isolating the affected systems, alerting security personnel, and launching remediation actions. Agility in this response minimizes the impact of any security breach and helps continuity in the telemedicine service.
5. Compliance and Regulatory Adherence: AI can help the telemedicine platform stay in full regulatory compliance. Automating compliance monitoring and reporting, AI keeps the habits of telemedicine in conformation to the likes of the United States' Health Insurance Portability and Accountability Act and the European Union's General Data Protection Regulation. Supporting audits, AI can provide very detailed logs and analyses of data access and usage, hence tending to transparent and efficient compliance management.
6. Better User Experience and Trust: AI in telemedicine security enhances user experience because it facilitates smooth and secure interactions. AI-driven security measures reduce disruptions to the service and ensure that patients and

healthcare providers feel confident using the telemedicine platform. By enhancing security and protection of patient data, AI builds trust and fosters further use of telemedicine services.

7. Future Research and Development: With increasing development in AI technologies, further research and development drive innovation in the security of telemedicine. Future developments that would most probably happen are sophisticated threat detection with advanced AI algorithms, better techniques that will help in preserving privacy, and integration of AI with emerging technologies like blockchain for safe data management. Collaboration by researchers, industry leaders, and regulatory bodies will be essential in overcoming new security challenges to ensure continued success with AI in telemedicine.

10.4 Ethical Considerations in AI-Driven Healthcare Security

Artificial Intelligence in healthcare security introduces massive improvements in safeguarding sensitive patient data and ensuring system efficiencies. However, it equally raises several ethical questions which must be met with due care to ensure the AI technologies are being used responsibly and with respect toward the rights of patients and society. It highlights some of the major ethical considerations of artificial intelligence-powered security in healthcare and points out considerations on how to cope with them [7].

1. Privacy and Confidentiality: Among the key ethical issues is how patient data privacy and confidentiality are maintained. Most AI applications require large volumes of personal health information for performing certain functions. The ethical challenge here is to keep this data safe from unauthorized access and misuse, and to ensure that AI technologies do not breach patient privacy. This protection should be highly secured through encryption and storage in a secure manner, and follow-through on related regulations such as HIPAA and GDPR. Moreover, it should be made clear to the patients how their data will be used, and they should have the right to opt in or out of this data sharing.
2. Informed Consent: AI application in healthcare security requires informed consent from the patient regarding data collection. The ethical approach demands that every patient fully understands how AI systems make use of their data, including risks and benefits that may be accruable. Communication needs to be transparent while consent to collect and analyze data must be clearly given to ensure trust and respect for autonomy.
3. Bias and Fairness: AI algorithms may further propagate an existing bias or exacerbate one if the training is based on biased datasets. In this respect, healthcare may result in disparate treatment outcomes and further propagate disparities across different patient groups. Fairness in AI-driven security requires proactive seeking and mitigation of biases within the training data and in algorithmic

decision-making processes in healthcare. For that reason, inclusivity and equity in AI designs should be promoted by researchers and practitioners while developing new models to avoid discrimination against some form of patient.

4. Accountability and Transparency: Applications of AI operate as black boxes, and very little can be interpreted of how certain decisions are arrived at. Such opaqueness inherently threatens to bring to a standstill accountability and trust. Ethics in deploying AI require the making of explainable AI models that shall provide an insight into how the decisions are reached and, therefore, make the healthcare professional and patients understand the output that comes out of these models. More importantly, clear lines of accountability need to be drawn on consequences and resulting actions related to AI-driven decisions. This is the only way issues can be addressed, and responsibilities discharged.
5. Ownership and Control of Data: As more and more patient data are collected and analyzed by these AI systems, questions regarding ownership and control arise. It is the right of the patients to own their personal health information and exercise control over its use. Ethical best practices range from putting in place clear policies on the ownership of data, access, rectification, and erasure by the patients, to the assurance that data is not used beyond the purpose for which consent was sought.
6. Safety and Risk Management: While AI is improving security, it is equally introducing new forms of vulnerabilities. Ensuring that AI-driven security mechanisms themselves are secure and resilient against attack is an ethical requirement. This involves periodic security audits and vulnerability assessments with strong safeguards to prevent potential breaches and misuse of AI systems.
7. Implications for Health Professionals: The integration of AI in health security could imply varied things in the jobs of health professionals. This concretely means that a need actually exists to ensure that ethics relevant to decision-making processes of AI result in diminished human oversight and reliance on automatic systems. Training and education are required in making sure that these health professionals can cooperate effectively with these AI systems and provide person-centered patient care at the same time.
8. Long-term Societal Implications: The wide acceptance of AI into healthcare security will have long-term implications on society, including but not limited to shifts in levels of power, changes in models of healthcare delivery, and impacts on patient-provider relationships. Ethical consideration covers rating and mitigating negative impacts on society, ensuring that AI technologies make positive contributions to the general healthcare ecosystem.
9. Ethics in Governance and Regulation: Stringent development of ethical guidance and regulation about the use of AI in health will help alleviate these issues. It has to be achieved by collaboration of researchers, policy makers, and ethicists who are developing standards and best practices that foster responsible use of AI while protecting patient rights.

10.5 Conclusion

With AI, much transformation has been enabled in healthcare security, whereby one can appreciate how much more promise lies ahead in further data protection of sensitive patient information, operational efficiencies, and quality care overall. These include among others: nodal areas of emerging threats in AI-enabled healthcare systems; integrating AI with blockchain for increased security; personalized security protocols; AI for assessment and management of risk; the future of AI in securing telemedicine; and a few other ethical issues that are very important. Artificial Intelligence is truly capable of vast data analytics and pattern recognition, and this has changed the way healthcare systems respond to security challenges. Yet with this technology also come new risks and ethical dilemmas to address in the full capturing of its potential. The emergence of new threats, such as adversarial attacks, data poisoning, and insider threats, is evidence of continued innovation in security measures. The integration of AI with blockchain makes for a very encouraging approach: not only for improving data integrity, but also for transparency. Thus, personalized security protocols ensure protection by matching up needs and behaviors at the level of the individual. AI is therefore very bright in the future of telemedicine security, as it enhances threat detection, data privacy, and compliance with the regulatory standards. Again, such ethical considerations regarding privacy, bias, transparency, and ownership of data are of prime importance, while their imperatives for responsible implementation and good governance must be underlined. In all, this roadmap to an efficient and secure health environment using AI stands on one variegated pathway that treads the judicious middle between technology advancement and ethical concern. Future threats will be averted or reduced to a minimum, while innovative integrations will be embraced, and principles upheld during the creation of resilience in healthcare systems, offering security for patient data, efficient service delivery, and building trust. To continue developing AI, ongoing research and collaboration, together with informed deployment, will be required to visualize a future where AI operates in servicing not only the security of healthcare in new dimensions but also in maintaining the highest levels of ethics and care practice.

References

1. khan, B., Fatima, H., Qureshi, A. et al. Drawbacks of Artificial Intelligence and Their Potential Solutions in the Healthcare Sector. Biomedical Materials & Devices 1, 731–738 (2023). https://doi.org/10.1007/s44174-023-00063-2
2. Kelly, C.J., Karthikesalingam, A., Suleyman, M. et al. Key challenges for delivering clinical impact with artificial intelligence. BMC Med 17, 195 (2019). https://doi.org/10.1186/s12916-019-1426-2
3. Tagde P, Tagde S, Bhattacharya T, Tagde P, Chopra H, Akter R, Kaushik D, Rahman MH. Blockchain and artificial intelligence technology in e-Health. Environ Sci Pollut Res Int.

2021 Oct;28(38):52810–52831. https://doi.org/10.1007/s11356-021-16223-0. Epub 2021 Sep 2. PMID: 34476701; PMCID: PMC8412875.
4. Hashmi, E., Yamin, M.M. & Yayilgan, S.Y. Securing tomorrow: a comprehensive survey on the synergy of Artificial Intelligence and information security. AI Ethics (2024). https://doi.org/10.1007/s43681-024-00529-z
5. Chen, SF., Loguercio, S., Chen, KY. et al. Artificial Intelligence for Risk Assessment on Primary Prevention of Coronary Artery Disease. Curr Cardiovasc Risk Rep 17, 215–231 (2023). https://doi.org/10.1007/s12170-023-00731-4
6. Camacho Clavijo, S. AI assessment tools for decision-making on telemedicine: liability in case of mistakes. Discov Artif Intell 4, 24 (2024). https://doi.org/10.1007/s44163-024-00117-4
7. Karimian, G., Petelos, E. & Evers, S.M.A.A. The ethical issues of the application of artificial intelligence in healthcare: a systematic scoping review. AI Ethics 2, 539–551 (2022). https://doi.org/10.1007/s43681-021-00131-7

Index

S. Gupta et al., *Artificial Intelligence-Enabled Security for Healthcare Systems*, https://doi.org/10.1007/978-3-031-82810-2

The manufacturer's authorised representative in the EU is Springer Nature Customer Service Centre GmbH, Europaplatz 3, 69115 Heidelberg, Germany. If you have any concerns regarding our products, please contact ProductSafety@springernature.com

Printed and bound by CPI Group (UK) Ltd, Croydon, CR0 4YY
30/09/2026
02225568-0001